MW01131931

The ultimate guide to

Low & Fluctuating

Blood Pressure

Causes, symptoms, home tests, and tips

Hypotension • white coat syndrome • pre-hypertension • atherosclerosis
• orthostatic hypotension • POTS • and more

Dr. Dorothy Adamiak, ND

LiveUthing Press

Cover design by Matthew Shepherd
http://ninjas.digital
Cover art © by Dr.D.Adamiak, ND
Editing by Alethea Spiridon Hopson
www.freelanceeditor.ca

ISBN-10: 1519398034
ISBN-13: 978-1519398031

Disclaimer
All information provided in this book is for educational purposes only. The information is not intended as a substitute for the medical advice of physicians. The reader should regularly consult a physician in matters relating to his/her health and particularly with respect to any symptoms that may require diagnosis or medical attention. This information is not intended to replace clinical judgment or guide individual patient care in any manner.

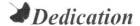Dedication

To Jack Canfield,

the author of "Chicken Soup for the Soul"

whose incredible story of success became my guiding light

&

To Steve Harrison,

speaker, author, and expert motivator

who persistently kept flooding my e-mails with mission reminders

It worked!

Thank You

A Note about the Language:

This book has been written for a reader without medical training.

If you are a health care provider you should know that simplifications and repetitiveness have been done on purpose in attempt to make health concepts accessible to a wider audience. Such simple, anecdotal, and free from medical jargon approach, has proven to be the most effective communication platform in my clinical practice.

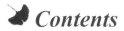 *Contents*

Small steps, big effects

More symptoms, tests, and tips

Because

Nothing is Random

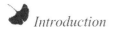 *Introduction*

Every book starts with a story….

For many years I had chronic fatigue syndrome. I was lifeless, depressed, and unproductive. My family doctor did all sorts of blood work, all of which turned out normal. I was pronounced "healthy." Meanwhile, I did not feel so. I could not hold a job, read a page without forgetting, and did not understand my woozy feeling in my head. I did not know why I felt worse after exercise and why exertion felt different to me than to other people. I worked hard, but my efforts were not rewarded by expected results. Everything felt hard, difficult, and tedious. Because of that I learned to procrastinate. I was slowly turning into a sloth.

It was frustrating. My doctor said I was "healthy" and suggested I would benefit from talking to a psychotherapist or maybe go on an antidepressant. Otherwise, there was nothing wrong with me. Despite health assurances, my life continued on a slow and wearisome path, nothing I would call healthy.

I took my doctor's advice and consulted a psychotherapist that said the same thing as my family doctor: "there is nothing wrong with you." So what now? Whom do I go to? Who can help? I was completely disappointed with my diagnosis. Since getting help was futile I decided to take my health in my own hands.

Totally frustrated, one day I got a strange idea: I am going to become a doctor myself. Either I will find a cure or my life would continue being miserable till no end. So I did. I enrolled in a four year accredited program to become a naturopathic doctor. I finished with top marks and got an official licensing number.

This was a great beginning. And although all the knowledge I gained through advanced schooling did not solve my chronic fatigue dilemma I did not give up. I felt I was close, but I had to put all the pieces of the puzzle together, and few were still missing.

My continuous interest in chronic fatigue led me to researching major health influencers: digestion and nutrition, immune system, hormones, nervous system, and eventually circulation. I was tireless and passionate about finding out the answers and eventually I got rewarded. Over the years I managed to put the missing health pieces together for myself and countless others.

Today, after gathering experience through two decades of clinical practice, attending countless courses, earning certifications and specializations, and sifting through a high-rise stack of research papers I know I can help you fast-track your own journey towards health.

So have a great read. Learn, discover, and get back to health. DrD

Meet DrD
YouTube: 2:21

https://youtu.be/9OhTkNuuRwU

Chapter 1

Three crucial health lessons

Do I have a heart disease? Is there something wrong with my blood pressure? Are circulatory changes an inevitable part of aging? If my dad had a stroke, does it mean I will have it too? Is there anything I can do not to end up with dementia, like my mom did?

You may have many unanswered questions, fear, and worry about health. I had those too in the past. I was riddled with anxieties and insecurities about my future. I was not sure if my body was healthy and if there was anything that could help me avoid my genetic fate.

I lost those fears for good. Today, having gone through thousands of patient files I am a firm believer that better health is within everyone's reach and the journey towards it is frequently simpler than assumed, regardless of whether it'll be battling headaches, reducing fatigue, reversing diabetes, or taming erratic blood pressure.

But getting healthier does not mean swallowing more pills for weight loss, cholesterol, or circulation. It means having a youthful, zestful, and functional body without having to take pills for controlling symptoms, lab values, and imbalanced physiology. A healthy body does not need health crutches. A healthy body maintains health by itself. It does not need pills to do so.

Yet prescribing pills for a condition is a common practice. There are pills for arthritis, blood thinning, psoriasis and three thousands other conditions. They are convenient and they work. The problem is that they work only temporarily, for a day or so… that's why you need to keep on taking them. If you don't your symptoms return, lab values get out of whack, and neither you nor your doctor is happy.

Getting back to health and getting unstuck from pills needs a different mindset. I've learnt many health lessons over the years and three of them I want to share with you today.

Lesson #1

Nothing is random. Headaches come from somewhere, diabetes has a cause, and high cholesterol is not a body error. Blood pressure is not any different. Even small dips and spikes in blood pressure show up for a reason; so do continuously high or low blood pressure patterns.

Lesson #2

Everything is connected. You can't have perfect blood sugar without a well-functioning liver, neither strong immune system without good gut flora. In order to keep blood pressure at a steady level you have to look beyond circulatory system and take digestion, hormones, and the nervous system into consideration.

Lesson #3

Many illness and diseases that are attributed to old age are actually not due to aging at all, but to a misguided lifestyle. You can halt degenerative processes, slow down aging, and reverse many ailments, including diseases of the heart, by making lifestyle changes.

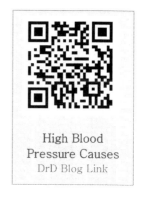

High Blood Pressure Causes
DrD Blog Link

http://goo.gl/oUCOLJ

Chapter 2

Worse than high blood pressure?

Low and fluctuating blood pressure numbers have never been hot topics. There are no bold headlines screaming loudly *"A new cure for LOW blood pressure found!"* or *"Science one step closer to finding a gene that causes FLUCTUATING blood pressure!"*

There is not enough drama in low blood pressure to raise eyebrows or cause a sense of urgency among health professionals. Many doctors see low blood pressure as neither a big problem nor an urgent concern to be treated. Low blood pressure in contrast to high blood pressure does not pose a lethal danger and thus rarely attracts attention. It is generally known that people don't die of *low* blood pressure. They die of *high* blood pressure.

Not so mild side of low blood pressure

It is *high*, not *low* blood pressure that is a dangerous killer, a source of strokes that can permanently cause damage or even take one's life within minutes. But low blood pressure is nothing like that. It is quiet, chronic, and annoying. One can live with it for a long time, so in a vast majority of cases the prescription for low blood pressure is limited to "monitoring" rather than "medicating."

Low blood pressure sufferers themselves are also not sufficiently alerted to its danger. Due to lack of alarming news, an easy-going approach of doctors, slowness of its progression, and long-term chronicity of blood pressure lows, those who have them think of low blood pressure symptoms more like an annoyance rather than a disease. A condition one can live with and a condition that is not dangerous enough to necessitate treatment.

However, behind a mild demeanor hides a sneaky health robber. This apparently mild condition, which is difficult to blame for any wrongdoing, can over time erode body vitality. Just like a river capable of eroding shores and flattening rocks, low blood pressure can do extensive damage to the body over time. It can lower vital capacity, reduce organ function, and even make permanent changes to the brain. Low blood pressure is not an innocuous, forget-about state. It is a concealed health hazard.

The frustration of lows and highs

Fluctuating blood pressure, a cousin of low blood pressure, requires special explanation. Fluctuating blood pressure happens when the numbers go up and down erratically and beyond normal limits. Blood pressure see-sawing is very confusing to many health practitioners. It is also difficult to manage and in my clinical experience it is seldom satisfactorily resolved with prescription medication.

Fluctuating blood pressure can be frustrating to doctors and patients alike. Stabilizing erratic blood pressure requires advanced medical knowledge and managing it with prescription drugs calls for incredible pharmaceutical finesse as well as substantial experience in cardiovascular medicine, not a combination every doctor possesses.

Fluctuating blood pressure is more exhausting to live with than low blood pressure. One has a much easier time to get accustomed to a steady state of low than to constant capricious blood pressure swings. Continuous blood pressure ups and downs can be annoying, unpleasant, and even frightful. Even worse, these fluctuations happen suddenly at any time of the day and night, making the person anxious and apprehensive to go out and participate in any activities whether it be something simple like walking or eating. Fluctuating blood pressure can be unpredictable and can keep the victims permanently homebound.

Fluctuating blood pressure is not only more difficult to handle than low blood pressure, but it also poses a much larger health hazard. Recent research suggests that erratic blood pressure, which was previously thought as banal, can be even more deadly than a steady state of high blood pressure, a well-acknowledged cardiovascular menace.

We are still years away from widespread public awareness about abnormal blood pressure changes and decades away from early diagnosing and impeccable treatment of this derailed health state.

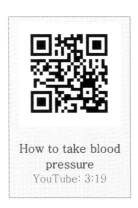

How to take blood
pressure
YouTube: 3:19

https://youtu.be/OwMR8ggkHXI

Chapter 3

Missing diagnosis

So you think there is something wrong with your blood pressure, but you also have other symptoms. You feel weak, spacey, fuzzy, and sort of drunk in your head. It makes you ponder: are your blood pressure and head symptoms in any way correlated or do you have two separate issues—a heart problem and head problem? Your doctor insists your blood pressure is good but can't figure out the source of the head symptoms. What a situation!

Motley of blood pressure symptoms

Let's un-confuse at least one thing for now: blood pressure symptoms. Low blood pressure symptoms are not the same for everyone and they can be so diverse that they can be mistaken for other health issues. It is not uncommon to misdiagnose them as digestive, respiratory, immune, or musculoskeletal ailments. Low blood pressure symptoms are not always limited to fatigue. They can also show up as shortness of breath, headache, stiff neck, cough, indigestion, and even forgetfulness.

ABC of Numbers

Chapter 4

So, what's normal?

What is normal blood pressure? What's below normal and what's fluctuating? Before we go any further you need to know some basic blood pressure rules.

A North American blood pressure ideal is said to be 120/80 mmHg, but that does not mean that anything different than that number is bad. In case you see different blood pressure numbers on the monitor don't panic. Normal blood pressure can vary significantly among individuals and even low numbers like 110/70 mmHg or high numbers like 130/84 mmHg should not cause a concern.

To simplify blood pressure math, current guidelines clearly divide numbers into normal, low, and high ranges. The rules are straightforward and easy to understand. However, before you start comparing your numbers to the chart keep one thing in mind:

Normal blood pressure varies between individuals and also fluctuates depending on circumstances.

When is it hypotension?

The guidelines state that blood pressure must fall below 90/60 mmHg for it to be considered low, or "hypotensive." But in order to get a "hypotension" diagnosis it is not enough to see these numbers once. However, even if you repeatedly see these numbers on your blood pressure monitor, your honest word will never be sufficient for a doctor, because these low numbers must be verified by a medical practitioner. After all a weak battery or a tube leak on your home pressure monitor can easily play tricks on the results. Your doctor has to see the numbers several times in his office to be concerned about low blood pressure as a condition.

Should it fluctuate?

Learning whether fluctuating blood pressure is normal or abnormal is not any different than checking for hypotension. Blood pressure fluctuates constantly and in order to correctly measure the amplitude of fluctuations your doctor may suggest monitoring with a Holter. A Holter is an automatic blood pressure monitor designed to inflate the cuff every few minutes. It does it even when you sleep.

Blood pressure fluctuations may be startlingly high. Did you know that an average healthy individual may increase his top (systolic) number by as much as 70 points during various activities? That sudden spike may be not only normal, but absolutely necessary during many heavy-duty efforts. Yet not all spikes are normal or healthy. The key to healthy heart is to distinguish between the good ones and the bad ones. How to separate healthy from unhealthy is a topic of the next chapter.

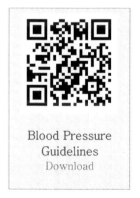

Blood Pressure
Guidelines
Download

http://goo.gl/OLBz4a

So what's your blood pressure on a daily basis? Carry the cuff with you and test blood pressure at different occasions: while listening to music, reading a novel, while chatting in a coffee shop, or sitting in a park while kids are playing. With this method you can see how your blood pressure behaves under various circumstances like while relaxed, bored, and maybe also hungry, or tired. Compare these numbers to the chart below. If something does not look right consult a health practitioner for further testing or advice.

So what's normal?

The chart below will give you a snapshot of the ranges for normal, low, and high blood pressure. These numbers apply to measurements taken at a normal *relaxed* state AKA *sitting*. The numbers do not apply when readings are taken during physical exertion or various activities. For example, you cannot use this chart for blood pressure taken while exercising or screaming while watching a horror movie.

		Top number (systolic in mmHg)	Bottom number (diastolic in mmHg)
☹☹	High blood pressure - extreme	Above 180	Above 110
☹	High blood pressure – stage 2	160 - 179	100 - 109
☹	**High** blood pressure – stage 1	140-159	90 - 99
🙂	Normal high (pre-hypertension)	139 - 121	81 - 89
☺	**Standard - normal**	120	80
🙂	Normal low	119 - 91	79 - 61
☹	**Low** blood pressure	Below 90	Below 60
☹☹	Low blood pressure – faint range	Below 60	

Chapter 5

Fluctuations that are good

There is a widely prevailing belief that healthy blood pressure should be steady throughout the day. After all, every doctor says it should be 120/80 mmHg, not 140/83 mmHg one minute, and 110/73 mmHg another time. Yet those who record their blood pressure several times a day are astounded to find out that their numbers vary every time they test. Some people are tempted to blame the fluctuations on the faulty monitor. Some worry and question the health of their heart.

But wait a minute! Should blood pressure be always 120/80 mmHg regardless whether you are sitting, sleeping, talking, or exercising? Should it be the same whether you are lifting, dancing, or relaxing? Not at all! In fact, if you find that your blood pressure is always 120/80 mmHg regardless of your activity you should be really, really concerned.

Blood pressure adjusts to activity

Did you know that physical activity, even as minor as talking or laughing, can cause noticeable changes in blood pressure? That's why when you measure blood pressure for assessment purposes you should not talk, laugh, or stand.

Blood pressure follows a simple principle: the more intense the activity, the higher the spike. Thus, walking should cause only a small change in blood pressure, while heavy exercise may really drive the numbers up. Weight lifters are known to register a spike in blood pressure as high as 480/350 mmHg during the time of extreme lifting feats.[1]

It's not hypertension!

Some years ago I had a case of a lady in her 60s. This Polish gal never exercised. As many women her age, culture and upbringing she thought exercise was a modern invention, a nuisance, and a complete waste of time. After all "she was always active and moving about." She was doing laundry, dusting, washing dishes, sweeping floors, and going grocery shopping. That was enough for her. She was firm about that.

She denied any heart or cardiovascular problems, but she was keen on health. She measured her heart health by checking her blood pressure, which was always the same at 110/70 mmHg. Her doctor told her to measure blood pressure while resting, so she did dutifully and she was always proud of her unchangeable numbers. She thus believed her heart was in peak shape and there was nothing that should be changed in that department. She insisted she was healthy with good blood pressure. She did not see a need to change anything, and she refused any talk about nonsense exercises.

The truth was that her heart was totally unfit. She needed exercise badly, but she did not want to hear about it. I nearly got grey with frustration. She needed to exercise to strengthen her heart, but she insisted the other way: her heart was good and her blood pressure was the proof.

We had long discussions on fitness, heart strength, and exercise. She did not budge. She never ran, lifted weights, played tennis, or did yoga. What for? Stupid exercises. These are for people who have too much time. She was too busy doing house chores. One day she agreed to prove me wrong about her fitness abilities and we proceeded with the test.

I put her on elliptical to measure her fitness level and at the same time hoped to prompt her that there could be room for improvement. The test was meant to be super easy, causal walking for ten minutes on the lowest level, nothing more than leg swinging.

She started hesitantly. She was anxious, awkward, and unwilling. She stopped at two minutes. She did not want to continue. I asked why? After a few minutes of listening to her nervous explanations I made out several reasons. She was afraid of exertion, after-pains, oxygen deprivation, potential injury, heart attack, falling off the machine, braking bones, and anything imaginable. There was no point to continue any further.

I checked her blood pressure at that time. It was 145/86. She panicked. She never saw it that high—145/86 mmHg is high blood pressure. OMG! Exercise gave her hypertension and now she may even get a stroke! Her heart was sick, exactly what she was afraid of. She would not exercise again. It was too horrifying to see those high numbers.

Know before panicking

This story was one of my earlier unforgettable lessons on how people understand cardiovascular health and how they interpret blood pressure numbers. Blood pressure monitoring can truly be a tremendous help in checking cardiovascular prowess, but you need to know a few things beyond 120/80.

Without knowing what's right, what's wrong, and what's normal it is easy to get lost in numbers, misunderstand and misinterpret the results. Regardless of whether your blood pressure is low, high, or fluctuating you need to know its details before making any conclusions.

Situation Specific
BP Log
Download

http://goo.gl/BIJYV1

It will take you approximately three days to do sufficient tests to get to know your individual blood pressure pattern. Do not compare your numbers to anyone else. Refrain from making definite conclusions about the results unless you read this book to the end. Take the measurements as they are and do not panic if they do not fit inside "healthy" ranges. Remember these healthy ranges apply only to measurement taken at REST, while SITTING.

Discover your own blood pressure pattern

Over the next few days you will be recording blood pressure behavior in various situations. Make sure your blood pressure monitor is fully operational, has all components working (no air leaks) and batteries are fully charged. These results will be most meaningful if you are not on any blood pressure medications. Blood pressure medications are designed to make blood pressure changes, so if you are taking them while doing the tests you will need a professional help in interpreting the results.

For example, if you registered 120/80 mmHg while taking anti-hypertensive drugs, it does not mean you do not have a hypertensive disease. It means that you have hypertension that is well controlled by medication.

To help with accurate analysis, record your meds, their dose, and timing in the box above the chart. Even if you are tempted to make the test most accurate, do not take yourself off any medication during test days. Sudden cessation of meds can destabilize your cardiovascular system, put you in danger, and make it harder to regulate your blood pressure afterwards.

Also be aware that meds take several days to leave your body. There will be enough drug residue over the next few days after stopping them to skew the results, so don't try to cheat.

Take the next three days to do the tests and fill out the chart below (or make your own chart). Take blood pressure measurements while *sitting*. Do not interpret the numbers as yet, just notice how they fluctuate. You will learn what these fluctuations mean a little bit later.

Drug/supplement name	Dose	Time(s) taken

Situation	Day 1	Day 2	Day 3
On waking, still in bed			
Before breakfast			
1 hr after breakfast			
Sitting quietly sometime between breakfast and lunch			
When you are about to take a nap			
1 hr after dinner			
Sitting quietly in the evening			
Right after strenuous heavy lifting			
When you are hungry			
Right after a long walk			
Right after a stressful situation			
Right after your regular exercise session			
Right after slow deep breaths for a minute			
At a doctor's office			

Chapter 6

Normal limits of ups and downs

The few days of taking blood pressure at different times may have been a real discovery. Did you find out that your blood pressure is never the same and that your numbers fluctuate more than expected? Soon you will find out whether this is a good thing or if you should be concerned.

You may have also noticed that your fluctuations are relatively predictable. They depend on the time of the day and what you were doing prior to testing. It made a huge difference to your blood pressure whether you ate, slept, exercised, or got stressed. Don't be surprised, but blood pressure may be quite unstable through the day. Blood pressure changes from minute to minute and there is a solid reason behind it.

It's all about oxygen

Changes in blood pressure are a must. They are healthy. They reflect the body's ability to adapt. A lack of fluctuation means that the cardiovascular system is "rigid" and does not move with the body. This is a bad thing. A steady blood pressure of 120/80 mmHg is seldom good, because increases and decreases in blood pressure during the day are not only normal, but actually reflect a healthy heart.

Think about it this way: increased physical activity requires more oxygen. During physical exertion muscles need sustained power. For that to happen muscle cells must get extra oxygen to produce energy. But how does the body get more oxygen? It does that by asking the heart to pump harder. When blood flows faster more oxygen is delivered.

But stronger heart beats mean higher blood pressure. That's nothing to be afraid of. That's good and that's healthy. Blood pressure should go up during physical exertion; otherwise you end up with an oxygen deficit.

Just as physical exertion depends on more oxygen, body stillness is happy with the opposite. A relaxed body requires less oxygen and that means the heart can take a break. Sleeping is the best example of body inactivity. Not surprisingly, blood pressure readings taken at night should register the lowest numbers.

No laughing matter!

Did you know that blood pressure is so responsive that mere talking can increases it? Laughter can also raise blood pressure, even as much as 15 systolic (top number) points[2]. You can measure the intensity of your laughter by checking your own blood pressure. Harder laugher makes blood pressure go higher.

First test your blood pressure while sitting relaxed. Then think of something funny and test your blood pressure. Laugh your hardest. The blood pressure increase reflects the power of your laughter. Traditional Chinese medicine says, "**joy fuels** the **heart**." So how much fuel do you have?

Now it makes perfect sense when your doctor insists not to talk or laugh while you take blood pressure. You don't want false readings, or worse a diagnosis of hypertension. Remember, there are no charts referencing blood pressure numbers while laughing. There are only charts for blood pressure while sitting and relaxing. Remember that when interpreting. Don't jump to erroneous conclusions. Avoid matching apples to oranges. Don't compare your blood pressure numbers during blood-pressure raising activities to the ranges meant for a relaxed state.

For adults only

If talking and laughing can bump the numbers up, would other activities do the same? What about washing dishes, sweeping floors, gardening or a common adult activity… sex? I did not find any studies on the first three, but since interest in sex is high, not surprisingly I found a few studies on that subject.

You may have already figured out that both males and females rely on a strong cardiovascular system for that unforgettable (for some) moment of sizzle. From your own experience you may recall a few cardiovascular give away clues: huffing and puffing, getting red in the face, and hearing the heart pounding. Females may get away by straining the heart only for that, but not males. Guys' sexual performance relies heavily on exclusive male sexual activator called a penis. And regardless who the partner is, a female, male, or a mirror, insufficient penile erections may be most embarrassing.

So how much blood pressure fluctuations should one have while romancing? It may be hard to believe, but there were quite a few studies done on frolicking couples. One of the studies was trying to establish even whether it makes a difference to blood pressure whether a man is on top or the bottom. A team of researchers set out to test blood pressure as well as various other parameters on couples enjoying each other while in different positions. This is the scoop:

Males in missionary position with normal heart function raised systolic blood pressure approximately by 20 mmHg points during intercourse. However, during an orgasm that number went up by 40 mmHg points. All observed men ended up beyond 160 mmHg regardless whether they were on top or the bottom while having fun.[3]

That's great, but why would you even bother to know that? Because if your blood pressure is generally "unwell" you may want to incorporate that knowledge into your daily life. Don't bother overthinking which sex position is better for your heart. It does not matter. Do what you like and feel free to enjoy.

But if your blood pressure is low and you need extra flow you may want to "schedule" sex during evening hours when blood pressure is naturally higher. Extra pressure makes the arousal easier and more voluptuous. Alternatively, if you have a tendency to high blood pressure you want to avoid that time.

Here is a side note on sex enjoyment. If you are on blood pressure medication you may experience arousal and erections differently. Penile inflation relies heavily on blood pressure and blood flow and many anti-hypertensive meds, because of their effects, can be problematic.[4] Out of all blood pressure medications diuretics seem to have the worst reputation. Up to one third of males receiving diuretics can experience decreased libido, erectile dysfunction, and difficulty ejaculation.[5]

Let's get physical!

If sex raises blood pressure would exercise do the same thing? In fact, it does. Hard working muscles need a generous supply of blood to perform well and for that reason any strenuous activity must increase blood pressure. Without the increase in blood pressure the muscles end up short of oxygen, tire out faster, and under-perform.

Shortage of oxygen can really wipe out physical performance. When deprived of oxygen mitochondria, our cellular power houses reduce their energy output from 32 to 2 units. This means if the blood pressure does not keep up with oxygen demands, the loss of physical power can be dramatic, going from 100% to 6% within seconds.

Every exertion needs blood pressure adjustment. A minor effort needs a smaller change, but a heavy exercise will push the heart to the max. While moderately exerting aerobic class usually increases blood pressure by 50-

70 mmHg points[6], heavy cycling, running, skating, or climbing can spike systolic to 180 mmHg. No need to panic. This is a normal reaction.

The most dramatic increase in blood pressure happens during weight lifting. Weight lifting, especially heavy leg presses, is capable of spiking blood pressure by more than 100 points. It is not unusual to register blood pressure numbers such as 230/250 mmHg or 255/190 mmHg in body builders during exercise.[7] Although tolerable by some, such dramatic spikes may not be endured in many untrained individuals, so size your weights accordingly.

Strenuous activities need blood pressure surges. These supply oxygen and give sufficient power to the muscles. However, elevated numbers *without* physical exertion is not to be considered a sign of good health.

Before deciding whether a blood pressure spike is appropriate or not, first consider the muscle factor. Blood pressure increase during physical exertion is a normal and necessary part of a well-functioning cardiovascular system, but blood pressure fluctuations while relaxed and sitting quietly are not.

White coat stress

You may have been wondering: should blood pressure go up when you sit at the doctor's office? It shouldn't, but when it does we call it "white coat syndrome." White coat syndrome is a name given to an excessive rise in blood pressure during doctor's visit AKA person in a white coat. White coat syndrome is very common. It affects about one third of individuals.[8]

Although white coat syndrome is not considered to be a disease studies suggests that individuals who have it need to check their health more thoroughly. Despite a widespread belief that blood pressure spike at doctor's office is innocent, white coat syndrome is not innocent at all.

A ten-year follow-up study of "healthy" people with white coat syndrome showed that these individuals might be not so healthy after all. During the study close to 20% (one in five) of these individuals succumbed to some kind of cardiovascular event, which included two heart-related deaths.[9]

White coat syndrome and cardiovascular health are not on the same page. White coat syndrome is one of the examples of unhealthy blood pressure fluctuations and one of the potentially first warning signs of approaching cardiovascular trouble.

But here is the good news. Naturally (not due to meds) occurring low blood pressure has the lowest probability of a white coat syndrome and the lowest risk of heart-related adverse events.

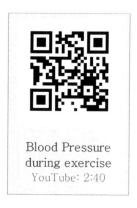

Blood Pressure
during exercise
YouTube: 2:40

https://youtu.be/ZLYzdbUHFMI

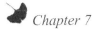 *Chapter 7*

Life is not still, your blood pressure isn't either

Are you then off the hook if blood pressure is good when a doctor checks it? Is the heart healthy if there are no signs of white coat syndrome and blood pressure numbers are in check?

In the previous chapters I asked you to take blood pressure measurements in various scenarios. Comparing blood pressure numbers during different situations may have led you to some discoveries.

For example, you could have found out that your numbers keep very low during exercise, which somehow correlated with breathlessness and feelings of exhaustion. Or maybe you discovered that the numbers shot up way high after a fiery disagreement with your spouse and the spike correlated with getting a massive headache afterwards.

These new personal findings beg a question. If your doctor checked your heart and said your blood pressure is good should you be concerned about your own findings discovered during the detective work? Should you in any way be in position to question your doctor's verdict of your cardiovascular perfection?

People make errors. Doctors make errors. Life is not still. Did you know that as many as 40% of people diagnosed by doctors as having normal blood pressure may actually have hypertension?[10] Blood pressure testing still does not reflect blood pressure whereabouts while actually living.

Find hidden clues

Ill-timed blood pressure fluctuations, which show up initially only during stressful situations, e.g. during a quarrel, tight deadline, or doctor's checkup are hidden signs of health changes. Studies are very clear that excessive spikes of blood pressure during excitement, such as mentioned earlier white coat syndrome, are correlated with increased risk for cardiovascular disease as well as diabetes.[11] But to detect these hidden spikes you need a more thorough testing that goes beyond a yearly medical checkup.

Nobody doubts that we have a massive hypertension epidemic. Yet somehow despite medical vigilance and focus on public awareness, many victims miss their early warning signs. The reason is simple. Most people check their blood pressure when still and not while living. However, moments of excitement are exactly when the first signs of unusually fluctuating blood pressure can be spotted.

I bet you`ve never checked blood pressure while watching a comedy, feverishly working overtime, or yelling at your kids. Nobody does. Yet, by measuring blood pressure exactly at these times you can detect early cardiovascular changes and have ample time for correction. Do not count on your medical doctor to alarm you to those hidden trouble spots. He cannot see them if he limits his observations to tests at his office. And this is frequently the case.

The current medical system is disease and not health-oriented. It is not interested in minor health changes, but in serious diagnosable conditions. Doctors treat disease, not minor health nuisances and diagnostic guidelines reflect that. For example, current Canadian guidelines state that if a doctor tests blood pressure and it is in pre-hypertension range (e.g. at 135/87 mmHg) he is advised to re-test it again only a year after.[12]

But what if you have a stressful job and blood pressure is constantly 160/95 mmHg Monday to Friday, and normal while off work? What if you are going through a divorce and meeting the spouse causes systolic spike beyond 200? Would checking your blood pressure only while relaxing and not while "living" make you any healthier and prevent you from getting a stroke?

If you limit yourself to only checking blood pressure while sitting quietly you may miss vital information about your heart: whether it responds property to physical exertion and whether it can "keep cool" in stressful situations. Not knowing how your cardiovascular system behaves under physical and emotional pressure may give you a false impression of being in good health. This should matter to you.

Blood pressure behaviour is an incredible reflection of health. Perfectly self-adjusting blood pressure is an indicator of well-functioning and well-synchronized nervous and cardiovascular systems. Permanent derailment in blood pressure is not something that happens overnight. Cardiovascular decompensation is slow progressing and it starts with occasional increase in blood pressure without physical exertion.

To manage health or disease?

Our current medical system focuses on detection of advanced degenerative processes called a disease, which appear only after years or decades of slowly declining health. Once the body reaches the disease phase reversing it is not easy. It takes much more effort to reverse already advanced degenerative processes and re-establish a healthy homeostasis then when the degenerative process has just started.

Be aware that not being diagnosed with a cardiovascular disease is not the equivalent to having impeccable cardiovascular health. It takes many years to go from perfect health to a degenerative disease that is ready for a diagnosis. To complicate matters, doctors are lacking tools to detect various stages of health before degenerative process is obvious. There are no cardiovascular reference ranges for perfect, good, average, or poor health. Doctors only have reference ranges for disease.

How is that information useful to you? What if you just want something simple? What if you just stick to taking blood pressure at rest? Is that wrong? No, it is not, but you need to be clear what information you want from the tests. If you are interested in finding out whether you have a diagnosable hypertensive disease testing blood pressure at rest only is sufficient. If you are interested in perfecting your cardiovascular and nervous system you should know the behaviour and fluctuation of your blood pressure at various times, at rest as well as while under stress. Checking blood pressure at rest will help manage hypertensive disease. Checking your blood pressure at different times will help manage cardiovascular health.

Do you have WCH?

WCH is an acronym for a special condition: Well Controlled Hypertension. I invented it to clarify a few things among patients. You won't find it in any medical dictionary or any textbook. Wiki doesn't have a page on it either. The reason for its invention is simple. I have met quite a few patients that benefited from that name.

One of them was Joseph, a 67-year-old Italian man. He insisted that he did not have hypertension even though he was on several anti-hypertensive medications. He insisted that he did not have high blood pressure, because his blood pressure was good. He checked it daily, so there was no error.

He understood that once his monitor did not show high numbers he was free of heart disease. His cardiovascular math was simple. His blood pressure was normal. Always. Even on his friend's machine. He checked. He did not want to have a heart disease. That's why he was taking the meds. Blood pressure monitors cannot all lie just like that. He got cured. Period.

There was no use for any discussion. Joseph was sure that his heart was in peak cardiovascular shape and hypertension was a thing of the past. He did not want to hear that drugs he was taking were only controlling the heart numbers and were masking the disease he still had. There was none of that.

I had to concede and this is when I came up with WCH. WCH filled the gap. It made Joseph feel better as he no longer had to worry about whether he was correct or not about hypertension. His wish was granted. He no longer had it. He just has WCH.

If you like that name, please use it. It means that the meds make your blood pressure monitor show healthy numbers. Tell your doctor about this. He may like the name as well.

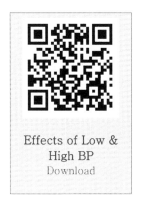

Effects of Low &
High BP
Download

http://goo.gl/shTLJ5

Chapter 8

Cardiovascular road map

If you read the previous chapters attentively you know that blood pressure fluctuations are common and their timing as well as amplitude can be used as an indicator of cardiovascular stability.

There are many stages between perfect health and disease. Monitoring blood pressure can help with that distinction, because inappropriately fluctuating blood pressure is one of the first signs of compromised circulation. To help you understand what happens with blood pressure as it goes through various health phases I divided them into nine stages.

Stage 0: Cardiovascular perfection

Normal blood pressure is registered at rest and during emotional stress; normal fluctuations are registered during physical exertion. Blood pressure returns to normal shortly after an activity is stopped.

Stage 1: Occasional spiking

Blood pressure numbers are normal with an exception of an occasional spike at an extra stressful situation such as visit at a doctor's office, after a massive dispute, during tight deadlines, and before a stressful job interview; otherwise, the body will continue having normal or slightly more intense blood pressure fluctuations during bouts of physical exertion; *white coat syndrome* may or may not be diagnosed and it may be the first and the only measurable sign that cardiovascular and nervous systems are starting to go in the wrong direction.

Stage 2: More frequent spikes

Frequent blood pressure elevations can be registered with commonly occurring life-stressors such as tiredness after work, mild disagreement with parents, after an exciting hockey game, after a short bus catching sprint, while driving in heavy traffic, etc. Daily blood pressure spiking means that the body's ability to deal with normal life events has been diminished. This is where measuring blood pressure at various activities is crucial, because even though cardiovascular health has already been compromised, blood pressure at rest may remain completely within normal limits.

Stage 3: Normal-high most of the time

Blood pressure does not seem to be going down to the ideal numbers or normal-low ranges like before and it seems to be a slightly elevated most of the time. Not enough to be alarming, but enough to keep a doctor on a watch guard. This in-between stage is the *final stop before an official diagnosis of hypertension.*

Stage 4: Diagnosis of hypertension

Blood pressure has edged towards hypertensive range and does not seem to want to go down regardless if you take it easy, sleep, or take vacation. It is time for an official *diagnosis of hypertension* and *first anti-hypertensive meds*. Once on them, blood pressure will settle down a little bit and the fluctuations will be less pronounced, but that effect will last only temporary, because blood pressure pills return neither heart nor blood vessels to health. They only help lowering high blood pressure. Do not assume that blood pressure medication will reverse hypertensive tendencies. For that you need major lifestyle changes.

Stage 5: Doubling up on meds

Since the first prescription medication wore off and is no longer effective it is time for another medication. By now it is clear that blood pressure meds only control, but do not cure hypertension and unless you are determined to reverse hypertension with lifestyle changes consider being stuck with the pills for good.

At this stage you may notice a disturbing trend. Despite the addition of the new medication, fluctuations of blood pressure can be seen as somehow more pronounced. New symptoms start showing up such as fatigue and weird unproductive cough. Anxiety may also be getting more noticeable.

Stage 6: Maximum intervention

At this stage blood pressure control requires a combination of several medications otherwise it keeps too high. The effect of continuous intake of meds and lack of sufficient measures to restore health is now catching up. Frequent bouts of fatigue are normal parts of life. General lack of energy and stamina is deepening and an overall feeling of wellness is leaving. Fluctuations of blood pressure now vary a lot between individuals and are greatly dependent on combinations of meds as well as depth of pathology.

Stage 7: Pronounced fluctuations

Despite several well-chosen prescription meds, blood pressure starts doing funny things. It goes up too high and then goes down too low. It is really difficult to keep it at a normal level. The gap between the top and the bottom numbers is widening as well. Instead of normal 40 point difference, it stretches up to 60, 70, and even 100 points at times. The feeling of wellness is now scarce. Weakness and lack of motivation is more pronounced. Mental confusion starts setting in.

Stage 8: Blood pressure pendulum

Blood pressure is getting really difficult to manage. The fluctuations are like pendulums going between highs and lows. Changes to medications make only a small difference. Blood pressure frequently goes to such lows that it evokes dizziness and instability. Forget about physical rigor. Any exercise poses a serious peril.

Stage 9: Oops!

Fluctuating and low blood pressure is now a normal part of life. Their effects are disastrous as even walking feels unsafe due to circulatory capriciousness. Dullness and mental confusion are noticeable to everyone. It is the phase when many victims become home-bound due to their physical and mental instability. Many would require supervision and help with daily tasks.

Think lifestyle, not pills

Wider fluctuations of blood pressure with noticeably higher highs and deeper lows are a natural consequence of advancing cardiovascular pathology. They are a giveaway that degenerative processes continue making progress. As blood vessels narrow, harden and become less elastic, they lose the ability to relax and expand. Stiff arteries are less capable of buffering heart beats and thus they produce a large gap between the top and the bottom blood pressure numbers.

Fluctuating blood pressure does not only signify problems with circulation. Fluctuating blood pressure is also linked to lower mental performance and poorer mood. It is also linked to some diseases like diabetes, ADHD, dementia, and Parkinson's.

Unless you decide to make changes to your lifestyle to reverse arterial deposits and bring back elasticity, your blood pressure will continue doing odd things. Re-elasticising blood vessels is not impossible, but it requires a significant change in lifestyle, commitment, and patience.

Be aware that excessive spikes in blood pressure are not an inevitable part of aging. Studies of different cultures show that increase in blood pressure is not related, as commonly thought, to aging but it actually ties in to lifestyle.[13] It is time to stop blaming time for its ill-health effects and look at our health habits. Advancing in age should lead to health wisdom, and not to illness and frailness.

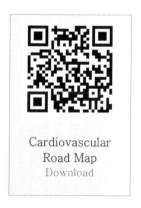

Cardiovascular
Road Map
Download

http://goo.gl/0HBnfZ

Is it Me or

Is it my Heart?

Chapter 9

The effects of long-term lows

I dedicated last few chapters to fluctuating numbers and now it is time to talk about low blood pressure. After all, in many cases hypotension is a part of a fluctuating pattern.

You may have noticed while studying nine cardiovascular stages explained in the previous chapter, that some phases include quite a bit of lows. However, these lows are not necessarily always a part of progressing cardiovascular decline. Many lows may be brought about solely by blood pressure reducing medication.

If you experience lows yourself, before going any further, you need to carefully evaluate where they come from. Make a clear distinction if these lows are naturally occurring fluctuations or fluctuations artificially induced by meds. This distinction will help you with their correction. Artificial lows in contrast to natural lows need adjustment to anti-hypertensive drugs, not a separate treatment.

If your blood pressure monitor shows low numbers do not leave the matters alone. Regardless of whether the lows are induced by medication or are your own, they have the same negative effect on the body.

Low isn't safe anymore

The innocence of hypotension is now coming into question as low blood pressure has been shown capable of eroding health. Studies pointed out that although hypotension is not as deadly as hypertension, it does have a substantial long-term adverse impact on our well-being. Low blood pressure contributes to poor circulation and reduces oxygen supply. Cold hands and feet are common example of those, so is foggy thinking at 90/50 mmHg. But these two easily spotted phenomena are not the only ones and are not the most worrisome.

Poor brain circulation and poor brain oxygenation have a much more profound effect on our lives than previously thought. Hypotension can negatively affect many areas including brain, mood, kidneys, senses, and life span. Even minute falls in blood pressure, falls that most doctors would dismiss as normal, have been found to have negative consequences.

Below are examples of heart effects that can be attributed to insufficient brain oxygenation:

- **Sensory impoverishment**: reduction in hearing and eyesight; this may manifest as bumping into things, tripping and falling, being prone to accidents; not hearing warning noises e.g. approaching car, sirens, and screams
- **Shift in demeanor**: personality changes, increasing anxiety, anger, and poorer interpersonal relationships; this may manifest as quarrelsome, inflammatory, conflictual personality
- **Loss of coordination**: difficulty with balance and movement; this may manifest as banging into things, slamming, hitting or dropping items
- **Visual impairment**: blurry vision, tunnel vision; this may manifest as difficulty reading signs, computer screens or newspapers
- **Communication issues**: slurring of speech, mispronunciation, difficulty forming sentences; this may manifest as dislike for participating in conversations and expressing self

- **Confusion**: exhibiting poor judgment, making wrong decisions; this may manifest as carelessness e.g. spending money unwisely or taking wrong turns while driving
- **Impairment of comprehension**: memory loss, forgetfulness; this may manifest as inattention e.g. missing a doctor's appointment or misplacing things
- **Bodily symptoms**: headaches, stiff neck etc; this may manifest as experiencing puzzling symptoms without any perceived cause

Pay attention to your body symptoms, because they may be your only clue as to blood pressure inappropriateness. Be keen on detecting low blood pressure numbers yourself, because your doctor may be interested in high blood pressure alone.

Hypotension reduces life success

From lower grades on math exams, to slower reaction times while driving, insufficient brain oxygenation can affect many aspects of life. Blood pressure decides whether you will have difficulty answering a question when confronted by a boss or can explain yourself when challenged by a family member. But low blood pressure is not only related to various levels of impairment in perception and cognition, but it also affects mood.

People with low blood pressure are found to have reduced motivation, increased feeling of hopelessness, and are less likely to put in any effort.[14] Anxiety, depression and aftereffects of low brain oxygenation may have far-reaching consequences at work and at home. They can lead to poorer interpersonal relationships, loss of satisfaction, higher stress, and lower productivity.

Depression, dementia, glaucoma, and life span

Low blood pressure effects are not limited to poorer brain oxygenation. Hypotension lowers oxygen delivery to vital organs and decreases organ function. Think about its effects on the liver, kidneys, bone marrow, or muscles. All organs are dependent on blood flow and the effect of diminished perfusion can have various consequences. For example, reduced blood flow to the liver can lead to slower drug detoxification and poorer blood flow to muscles can lead to weakness and meager performance at the gym.

Knowing your blood pressure whereabouts is essential, because studies point out that hypotension the increases risk for developing specific health problems. Here they are:

- Increased chances for **depression** and **anxiety**. A very large 2007 study done on over 60 thousand subjects found that regardless of age people with chronic low blood pressure are significantly more prone to depression and anxiety[15]
- Increased risk for **dementia**. Difficulty thinking, memorizing, and impaired cognition is a well-known short-term effect of blood pressure drop, but a recent study involving close to one thousand participant pointed out that long term insufficient blood perfusion is found along *permanent* changes to the brain. Even arrhythmia (skipping beats) which results in temporary minor lowering of blood pressure can cause deep changes in white matter of the brain.[16]
- Increased risk for **glaucoma**. A small study correlated reduction of visual field with low nighttime blood pressure. It turns out that the lower the dip during sleep and the longer its duration the higher the chances for visual loss. This visual impairment happens regardless whether the dips occur spontaneously or is induced by medication.[17]

- Decrease in **hearing** acuity. As per a research done at University of Bologna, Italy, hypotension can be blamed for hearing loss even in younger individuals. This 1999 study found that people with blood pressure below 105/60 mmHg have more than twice the risk for hearing impairment than people with blood pressure above these numbers.[18]
- Onset of ear noises, **ringing in ears**, and vertigo.[19, 20]
- Increased risk for **kidney failure**. Reduction of blood flow can damage any organ whether brain, heart, or kidneys. Recent studies show that acute kidney failure is typically preceded by an episode of low blood pressure.[21]
- Increased mortality in **infants** as well as their delayed motor development and hearing loss.[22]
- Shortened **life span**. An older 1989 study pointed out that not only high blood pressure, but also low blood pressure correlates with shortened life-span. In a group of elderly men with hypertension, low diastolic blood pressure increased, not decreased, their mortality and paradoxically higher diastolic numbers predicted survival.[23]

Slower beats, longer life?

While researching heart function and longevity I have found yet another interesting correlation. This one does not directly involve blood pressure, but rather heart rate. Don't be overly preoccupied by the findings, though. Treat them more like fun facts rather than predictions written in stone.

A paper written by June Liu and published in *Undergraduate Journal of Mathematical Modelling* in 2011 has pointed out a significant inverse relationship between human longevity and heart rate.[24] Apparently, people with slower heart rates have longer lives and people with the slowest heart live the longest.

The study concluded that people with an average heart rate of 70 beats per minute have an average life expectancy of 70 years. Those with faster heart rate can expect shorter lives. For example, people with heart rate of 90 per minute can reach a statistical lifespan of only 55 years. People with heart rate of 60 should reach an average of 82 years and people with 40 beats per minute can celebrate a fantastic 123 years.

Before grabbing your wrist to find the pulse be aware that this statistics may apply only to naturally occurring heart rate, which is not altered by medications.

If your heart rate is a bit on a high side, don't panic. Find a way of reducing it, either by learning how to cope with stress better or by increasing cardiovascular conditioning. Regardless of whether the numbers are true or not, superior emotional and physical fitness are always good health assets.

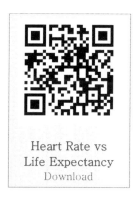

Heart Rate vs
Life Expectancy
Download

http://goo.gl/RIZK5l

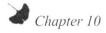

Chapter 10

Diagnostic limbo

In good medicine things are never wishy washy. Either you have something or you don't. There is no in between. Either you have diabetes or you don't. Either you have osteoporosis or you don't. Things are definite and for a reason. It helps doctors make proper decisions.

Doctors cannot treat patients for non-existent conditions. It is reasonable to think that a doctor cannot treat Alzheimer's if there is none, and cannot treat hearing loss if you hear well. Things are not any different with blood pressure. Before any treatment begins there has to be a diagnosis. But here is a trick. The current medical system recognizes only high or low blood pressure. There is nothing in between. Your doctor can treat you either for "hypertension" or "hypotension," but not for normal, normal-low, or fluctuating blood pressure. If you fall in those latter, you are out of luck.

In previous chapters you learned that hypotension and hypertension are not arbitrary numbers. You have hypertension if your blood pressure is consistently above 140/90 mmHg and hypotension if it is consistently below 90/60 mmHg. If you ended up with diagnosis of high or low blood pressure you will be treated accordingly. But what if you are somewhere in between?

Low blood pressure underestimation

Low blood pressure is easy to miss. Even though it has many negative effects countless people are allowed to walk about with untreated hypotension risking falls, dementia, eyesight, and hearing loss.

This under-recognition is not on purpose. There are many reasons for it. Firstly, health care practitioners see low blood pressure as a lesser health burden then high blood pressure, so the focus is on detection and treatment of highs, not lows. Secondly, low blood pressure is frequently masked by a temporary pressure increase due to excitement while at the doctor's office, so low blood pressure is seldom confirmed by clinicians during the physical exam time. Thirdly, there is not any simple and gentle pharmacological treatment for hypotension. The existing drug protocol for low blood pressure is reserved for more serious cases.

Improving odds for better health

Lack of diagnosis of hyper- or hypotension does not equal to living free from symptoms. Given the factors above it is not unimaginable that many people live with blood pressure numbers negatively affecting their mood, energy, and productivity. Some unfortunates may even be treated separately for depression, hearing loss, and dizziness and subject to ingesting numerous useless pills while the real cause of the problem remains hidden and is left untreated.

But lack of diagnosis does not mean you have to "live with it." There are many things you can do even if you are lacking the sympathetic ear of a doctor. The remaining part of this book will teach you a few neat home tests for the heart, explain other conditions your blood pressure may "qualify you for," and how to prevent and treat symptoms of dropping blood pressure.

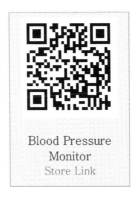

Blood Pressure
Monitor
Store Link

http://goo.gl/BkoV6j

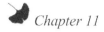 *Chapter 11*

Patterns of the heart

There is one more reason why detecting low blood pressure is difficult. Not everyone will have steady low blood pressure throughout the day. Many people experience isolated episodes of hypotension precipitated by specific activities (such as standing up), prompted by specific environmental triggers (e.g. rainy weather), or just occurring at a specific times (e.g. before menstruation).

There isn't any universal blood pressure mold everyone fits into. Everyone's heart is different. That's why understanding your own blood pressure pattern is vital. Knowing the details can prevent the confusion whether you have or don't have hypotension-related symptoms and give you a clearer idea about the underlying causes of blood pressure changes.

Have a keen eye

To familiarize yourself with your own pattern analyze the blood pressure log you filled out earlier. To gain even more knowledge about recurrence of the fluctuations, you may even create a completely new log with much more extensive situational checks. The more detailed checks and the more meticulous record keeping the better you'll be able to understand your pattern and correlate your symptoms to actual blood pressure readings.

I had numerous patients that took blood pressure medication faithfully without any intermittent check between doctor's visits. They were completely unaware of the possibility that their symptoms such as fatigue, headaches, and confusion may be due to missed blood pressure dips. After all, their doctor was treating them for high blood pressure, so low blood pressure was not a foreseen possibility.

Only a meticulous log can make blood pressure fluctuations evident. If you found a lot of lows, but your doctor gave you a diagnosis of high blood pressure you need to bring your findings to his attention. He did not give you wrong medication. He just needs to adjust it.

Keeping a blood pressure log is a must. Without a log you and your doctor may by puzzled as to why you're experiencing a never ending list of symptoms despite well-chosen prescription medications.

Food for
fluctuating BP
Download

http://goo.gl/zUmCl1

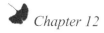

Chapter 12

Hypotensive personality

Is there something like a low blood pressure personality? One may argue that there is and may especially be expressed in those people for whom hypotension is a permanent feature of life.

Low blood pressure can contribute to low oxygenation and produce typical foggy brain symptoms: decreased ability to comprehend, memorize, and think. What follows are poor school grades, low productivity at work, and physical "laziness."

Feeling tired, acting placid, and demure is typical for people whose lives have been taken over by hypotension, but an exit from a "pushover" and "failure" may be just as easy as increasing the numbers. Many times when blood pressure normalizes the "losers" and "wimps" magically turn into intelligent, smart, and gutsy folks.

Personality makeover!

Maybe you can recognize your or someone else's traits from the list below. If so, there is a good chance that these traits may have something to do with blood pressure irregularities.

- **Apparent dullness**: Slow thinking, difficulty in understanding reading material, dullness that may be perceived as confusion or lack of comprehension

- **Unsteadiness**: Feeling of spaciness, whooziness, lightheadedness that reduces physical confidence and prevents experiencing full physical potential
- **Mental weakness**: Difficulty learning, trouble with focus and concentration; kids may have poor grades and dislike school
- **Anxieties**: Lack of zest for life, fearfulness, lack of confidence, sadness and depression; lack of motivation and general dissatisfaction with life for no discernible reason
- **Physical weakness**: Fatigue, dislike for exertion, apparent laziness, slow reactions that keep many from enjoying the more adventurous side of life
- **Frequent headaches**: headaches that are non-throbbing, but dull, pressing that are bothersome, but not bad enough to seek medical attention
- **Weird sensations in the head**: Ear pressure and fullness, humming in ears that is annoying but seldom diagnosed as problematic
- **Excessively delicate nature**: Paleness and loss of musculature, frailness, loss of vitality and poor blood flow
- **Symptoms of poor circulation**: Cold hands and feet, sensitivity to cold; fungal infections on toes as fungus thrives in areas with poor circulation
- **Aesthetic difficulties**: Poor quality hair, hair loss, hair dullness that can frustrate to no end; fragile nails

Wow! You may have just discovered that some symptoms and annoyances that may look "stuck on you" can actually be related to imperfections of cardiovascular physiology rather than inherent personality traits.

Although many personality traits remain unchangeable, traits dependent on cardiovascular performance can be modified. Gaining more control over the body in areas you may have given up hope is possible. Depressive tendencies, physical frailness, or weak mental performance can improve together with blood pressure numbers.

There is no point chasing supplements for anxiety, avoid physical intensity, or hide from the windy outdoors if all your body needs is better circulation. Take charge of your numbers and start living to your fullest.

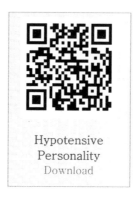

Hypotensive
Personality
Download

http://goo.gl/UiPAeQ

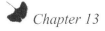 *Chapter 13*

Do you dip well?

Blood pressure does not stay steady flat throughout a twenty-four hour cycle. It has a natural diurnal cycle and the numbers have predictable circadian fluctuations. They keep higher during the day and go down at night.

This twenty-four-hour blood pressure variations attracted scientists' attention, who conducted studies to establish whether various diurnal patterns are in any way correlated with different levels of health. They found out that an average healthy person experiences a small drop of blood pressure while sleeping of a magnitude of about 10-20%.[25].Such a dip is a welcome sign of good health. Night should be a time for adequate rest also for the heart. Dips of a larger degree or a complete lack of dipping do not score well.

Things must go down overnight

By now it should be clear that healthy blood pressure never stays the same. Studies confirmed that certain fluctuations of blood pressure correlate with better health. Specifically, lack of overnight blood pressure dips can be seen as a warning for compromised health.

Studies correlated lack of blood pressure dipping with poorer sleep, night waking, and sleep apnea.[26] Non-dipping was also associated with enhanced risk of cardiovascular events[27] as well as endocrine and nervous system dysfunctions.[28] Non-dippers were found to be experiencing more stress, and have stronger family history of hypertension.[29] Remember, night dipping is one of those blood pressure fluctuations you *want to* have.

Lack of dipping at night is not a sign of good health, but inverse dipping, which an increase in blood pressure, is correlated with even worse prognosis. This paradoxical increase of blood pressure, called nocturnal hypertension, has been found to be present in a large proportion of people suffering from stroke.[30] Other studies also suggested that rise of blood pressure overnight is significantly related to poorer cardiovascular health. Some even proposed that an increase in systolic (top number) can be used as a predictor of approaching cardiovascular events.[31]

Dipping extreme

If dipping is good for a person with normal blood pressure, would dipping be in the same good category for a person who already has day-time low blood pressure? What if someone's daily average is around 100/70 mmHg or worse yet 95/62 mmHg? Would that someone end up faint or risk not waking up in the morning?

I am sure you had mornings that felt as if you haven't woken up. You felt tired despite spending all night long in bed apparently sleeping. If that happened once or twice you may disregard it, but if that is a frequent occurrence it is good to check what your heart is doing at night. Chances are that not being well rested in the morning simply means your oxygen delivery overnight has been compromised.

If you start low and have a small night-time dip you may still be fine, but what if you belong to a group of extreme dippers, people who get overnight blood pressure dips of more than 20%?[32, 33] What if you are one of those people who experience even more significant fluctuations, maybe in the range of 50 points? Would that cause harm?

Several studies have pointed out that extra low blood pressure at night isn't healthy. Even though low blood pressure in not considered a health hazard, research found that extreme lows can, just as the extreme highs, lead to cardiovascular events and brain damage.[34] People who register very low blood pressure overnight are prone to silent strokes[35] from insufficient blood flow to the brain.

These extreme dips are not good for the eyes either, as insufficient oxygen is capable of damaging the nerves and lead to vision loss.[36] People with diabetes and sleep apnea are frequently found among extreme dippers[37] so are people with a higher degree of arterial stiffening.[38]

Do you know your own night-time blood pressure pattern? For the above reasons you should. If you don't know how to go about it here is a solution: talk to your doctor to get you a Holter monitor, an automatic blood pressure measuring instrument. You will be instructed to wear it for two or three days. The Holter monitor will automatically check your blood pressure every few minutes and report the results to your doctor. If you, while wearing this monitor, also keep a log of your activities, the lessons you will get from analyzing the results may be invaluable.

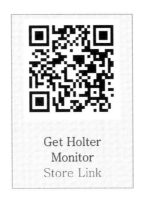

Get Holter Monitor Store Link

http://goo.gl/YY1TjW

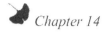
Chapter 14

Secrets of a zestful morning

Nine out of ten people do not know their blood pressure numbers.[39] Half of people with *high* blood pressure are unaware of it.[40] Barely anyone with low blood pressure know about their condition, and that's not because of lack of care.

Low blood pressure can easily get obscured because of natural blood pressure fluctuations. Many individuals experience dips of blood pressure intermittently throughout the day without having a clue about it.

I bet you don't roll out your blood pressure monitor when your eyes open in the morning and test your blood pressure before putting your feet on the ground. Very few people do. Obsessive testing in the morning is generally not a popular activity. Morning is a time of rush, not leisure, and can get really hectic if one has to go to work.

For most of us morning routines are efficiently shrunk to only essential procedures, which are usually devoid of optional health checks. Morning flow looks like this: wake up, pee, wash, beauty enhance, eat, and out to work.

Homemakers do things only with a slight modification: wake up, pee, wash, mirror check, drop kids off, back for breakfast and a mandatory nap if the night was crappy. The elderly, although not rushed by work schedule or kid duties, are haunted by their own peculiar time demon: physiological needs. Senior bladders don't wait and they need priority treatment. So regardless of life arrangements there is a slim chance that blood pressure gets tested in the early morning hours.

Tired, groggy, and dopy?

Mornings when you feel dopy, lightheaded, and dazed may suggest hypotension. But how would you ever guess that unless you get the monitor going right then and there to confirm the numbers? Without checking you may be tempted to blame the morning fatigue on a "restless" night and inclined to ignore the symptoms. You shouldn't. Lazy mornings can tell your hormonal health.

Morning awake

What comes down must go up. And so is the case with the blood pressure. In a healthy person the overnight dips are followed by day-time rises. The first anticipated blood pressure peak should appear soon after waking. The body needs it to face the day. It is exactly this blood pressure surge that transforms the morning from groggy to zestful. But what if you are one of those people who lack morning energy and rather spend an extra hour dozing off? You may be lacking in wakeup phenomenon.

The "get up" of blood pressure is largely determined by the amount of circulating cortisol. Cortisol not unlike blood pressure follows a twenty-four hour clock and also is inclined to fall overnight. This drop is good, needed, and necessary for well-being. Without it the body won't rest, because the release of cortisol is invariably followed by heightened alertness.[41] Cortisol increases blood pressure and prepares the body for action. This is why cortisol is called a stress hormone.

Cortisol's twenty-four hour cycle is rather predictable, but can change when health is compromised. In healthy individuals the lowest cortisol point occurs during the deepest part of the night, around 3 a.m. From then on it slowly goes up and peaks just before waking and then again shortly after that.

Three quarters of people are known to peak twice. The second peak taking place about twenty minutes after waking. This hormonal phenomenon, called cortisol-awake, is present in 77% of normal individuals.[42] Higher peaks appear in people who wake up easily, have good morning energy, and also experience blood pressure increase. In contrast, low peak, or a complete lack of, may not only mean low blood pressure in the morning, but also fatigue and pain.

Up, up but not too high

A person with a healthy cardiovascular system is supposed to experience a moderate blood pressure surge in the morning. Higher blood pressure flushes organs and delivers oxygen needed to face life stressors. Yet regardless of the circumstances this morning spike should never go above 140/90 mmHg.[43] Healthy and normal increases stay below that number.

Blood pressure spikes over 140/90 mmHg are seldom part of a healthy physiology. The highest number of sudden cardiac deaths is recorded in the morning hours, exactly when morning blood pressure peaks.[44] [45] Because blood pressure fluctuations correlate with cortisol levels[46] this rise of morning blood pressure is now being blamed on underlying hormonal variation, specifically excess morning cortisol.[47]

Don't panic! Although you may not know what happens with your morning cortisol, blood pressure checks upon waking are within your reach. It is worth knowing your morning blood pressure, not because it may be low, but also because it may be high.

Morning hypertension carries a risk. Its calculation is rather simple. For every 10 mmHg of increase in morning systolic (top number) above 140/90 mmHg, the risk of stroke goes up by 22%.[48] Excessive morning spikes are to be avoided for other reasons. They correlate with depression, dementia, sleep apnea, and metabolic syndrome.[49]

The appearance of low and high blood pressure in the morning is not a coincidence. Both are tied to the hormonal system and they are not without consequences. The good thing is that now you are in a better position to assess your disease risk just by checking blood pressure at a specific time of the day. Think about it this way: if you own a blood pressure monitor you own an incredible multipurpose assessment tool.

Cortisol flats

Too much cortisol in the morning is not good, but is low cortisol in the morning any better? For those who produce little of this energizing boost we may have to look beyond cardiovascular system and expand the investigation into cortisol production. Cortisol is produced by the adrenals and people with low morning cortisol may want to check those glands thoroughly. It is the mighty adrenals that orchestrate hormones and neurotransmitters needed for times of stress as well as times of Zen.

Weak adrenals are bad at their jobs. They do not produce sufficient cortisol for morning arousal. Suspect weak adrenals when you are unable to cope with stress, or when you feel nervous, anxious and apprehensive without a reason. Fatigued adrenals are not rare. They are common and they are known to turn a healthy, zestful, energetic morning into a lifeless, dull, and comatose drudgery.

But do not mistake adrenal fatigue with Addison's disease. These two cause constant confusion and misunderstanding between health professionals. Be aware that a conventionally trained physician will not be familiar with the concept of adrenal fatigue. He will only know Addison's disease. Asking your endocrinologist to diagnose adrenal fatigue will be futile. He cannot do it.

Addison's disease, which is the result of a complete exhaustion of adrenals, is relatively rare. It happens only in 1 in 20,000 people.[50] Addison's disease has straightforward diagnostic criteria that are easy to identify. A simple blood test will be sufficient to confirm adrenal's failure.

Both adrenal fatigue and adrenal failure (Addison's) will keep blood pressure low in the morning and likely also during the rest of the day. However, Addison's disease besides keeping blood pressure low can produce other symptoms, such as sudden body pains, low blood sugar, lethargy, or dark patches on the skin. By the time you have Addison's your health issues are obvious to everyone.

Addison's disease is an extreme far end of adrenal fatigue, but adrenals do not go from healthy to failing just like that. Between robust adrenals and Addison's disease the glands go through various performance stages ranging from sluggishness to weakness to exhaustion. Due to lack of established diagnostic ranges anything between normal-low and Addison's disease can fall into a category of adrenal fatigue.

Despite that diagnostic difficulty adrenal fatigue can still be established. But one cannot draw blood for that. Adrenal fatigue, in comparison to Addison's disease, is not diagnosed from a blood test, but from saliva samples. Four saliva samples collected during day-time hours are necessary to trace how cortisol behaves during the day. This saliva cortisol test may be "God-sent" for individuals who feel lifeless, tired, unmotivated, have consistently low or fluctuating blood pressure and don't know why.

In case you have the test done, hopefully in a reputable laboratory, I only have one request: do not run around with your report showing it to random health practitioners. The test results must be analyzed by an experienced clinician versed in endocrinology. Otherwise, you risk getting the wrong interpretation. Board-certified/licensed naturopathic doctors and doctors trained in functional medicine are generally familiar with various adrenal patterns including fatigue, weakness, exhaustion, and Addison`s disease. If you have access to such, establishing a relationship with one will be your best choice.

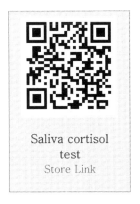

Saliva cortisol
test
Store Link

http://goo.gl/Jc2HBF

Small Steps

Big Effects

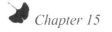 *Chapter 15*

Blood pressure levelling breakfast

Having a strong cortisol awake is only one reason behind higher blood pressure readings in the morning. What you have for breakfast is another.

Did you know that, depending what you eat, breakfasts can lower or increase the heart action? You may not care about that if your blood pressure is normal, but if your blood pressure is usually in the basement you may want to remember the tips below.

Did you hear that bananas have lots of potassium and are good for your heart? That is certainly true if you have hypertension, but not when you are battling with low blood pressure. Banana and milk cannot bless you with an energetic morning. Foods like banana and milk loaded with potassium and calcium can lower, but not increase blood pressure. Studies confirmed that there is a considerable inverse correlation between blood pressure and these minerals.[51] Both calcium and potassium have blood pressure lowering effects. The more of them the lower it gets.

Since banana and milk have a relaxing effect on cardiovascular system, don't use them when mornings already feel sluggish. Use them before bed to help with a good night sleep, or better yet, leave them for those with hypertension.

Coffee to the rescue

You may have also heard that coffee is bad and may have been tempted to avoid it for health reasons. But before you dump your java entirely consider that coffee can have an extraordinary morning wake up effect. This good wake up effect is believed to be at least partially due to coffee's ability to raise blood pressure. Hmm... but would that not give you hypertension?

Coffee and caffeine have been subjects of controversy for quite some time. Their effect on health and blood pressure has been studied extensively and verdicts were see-sawing from good to bad depending on the angle of the study.

When I learned that many of my low blood pressure patients dropped coffee out of their menu following the belief that coffee, just like pop or candy, is unhealthy I dedicated a few evenings to find out if their reasoning has any scientific basis.

Surprisingly, coffee and caffeine's effect on blood pressure has been well researched. The most interesting finding for me was that people with hypertension react differently to caffeinated beverages than people with normal blood pressure, and that younger people are affected more than older individuals. You see now that a doctor cannot just say coffee is good or bad for everyone, but needs to give advice tailored to health status and age of the patient.

Short-term vs. long-term

There is one more thing to consider. Coffee and caffeine is not just good or bad all the time, but they can have independently good or bad time-depended actions. One can divide the effects of caffeine into two categories:

- **immediate effect**, which reflects cardiovascular effect 30-60 min after ingestion and

- **long-term** which relates to drinking coffee regularly over many months or years.

Immediate effects are unequivocal: caffeinated coffee raises blood pressure, but how high the spike goes depends on the person's cardiovascular health. A study done in 2000 by a University of Oklahoma team found out that people with high or normal-high blood pressure numbers have the strongest reaction to caffeine. They respond to it with the highest blood pressure increase.[52]

The caffeine spike in people with normal blood pressure, in comparison to those with hypertension, is much smaller and also shorter-lasting. That means individuals with low or normal blood pressure should not worry that a cup of java could cause an immediate uncontrollable high blood pressure surge after consumption.

However, before adding coffee back to your breakfast, be aware that only real coffee with caffeine in it is capable of delivering this desired blood pressure boost, so forget about coffee substitutes or decafs. They won't do regardless of how much you like them and how much you think real coffee is a harmful substance.

One more thing. Are you on blood pressure medications? If yes, then even though you wake up with low blood pressure you actually belong to a category of people with high blood pressure. You don't have hypotension. You just ended up with a hypotensive *episode* due to poorly performing or inappropriately adjusted meds. In such case a java cup may need to be OK'd by your doctor first. But don't just avoid the brew because you are not sure or you don't want to bother the doctor. There are numerous benefits of drinking coffee that extend to many organs and systems, so if your cardiovascular system and your doctor is good with it, drinking coffee may be actually good for you.

Long-term effects of caffeinated coffee on blood pressure are a tad more obscure. There is still no consensus despite numerous studies on this topic. It can be quite baffling to learn that out of eighteen systematic studies five found no correlation between caffeine and blood pressure, six studies found positive correlation, and seven found inverse correlation between coffee drinking habits and hypertension. [53] As of today we are still not sure if long-term coffee consumption *causes* high blood pressure, but we can surely conclude that people with an already compromised cardiovascular system should be cautious with *excessive* coffee drinking habit.

Switching to tea?

Did you know that white, green, and black tea come from the same plant, *camellia sinensis*? Whether white tea becomes green or black is just a matter of timing of its harvest and further processing. For example green tea becomes black after being subject to oxidative fermentation. This process of changing color also changes taste, chemical composition, caffeine content and health properties of the leaves.[54]

We may be cautious about drinking coffee, but seldom anyone hesitates to drink tea due to its cardiovascular effects. Interestingly, a study done on green and black tea drinkers have shown that tea, despite a common myth of safety, is capable of producing a blood pressure spike as well. The spike that comes within thirty minutes after drinking may be substantial. Both green and black tea can cause such effect, but black tea usually causes higher blood pressure rises than green tea.[55]

Despite this surprising blood pressure spike, tea, whether green or black, does not seem to produce a long-term blood pressure effect, an effect which some studies suggest happens with coffee. Because of that long-term kindness, green or black tea may be a better choice for people with unstable blood pressure or people that are prone to hypertension. So if your cardiovascular system does not tolerate coffee, consider strong black or green tea as your morning blood pressure rising beverage.

Despite the findings, leave pop alone

Pop and energy drinks are also frequently used for a pick-me-up effect. Their caffeine content varies so does the blood pressure effect associated with it. Caffeinated sodas are capable of a blood pressure spike, but would caffeine in these beverages have the same effect as that found in tea or coffee?

Apparently, the blood pressure effect of pop is not only dependent on caffeine. It also depends on whether soda is sweetened with sugar or artificial sweetener. A ten-week experiment with pop drinkers brought an unusual discovery. Participants who drank sugar sweetened pop saw an increase in blood pressure. In contrast, those who consumed artificially sweetened soda registered lowered numbers at the end of the study.[56]

Sorry to say, but artificially-sweetened soda will not be prescribed for treatment of high blood pressure despite these findings. Habit of drinking pop correlates with poor nutrition, so do not expect pop to suddenly appear next to Hawthorn berries and aged garlic in a health food store isle.

This study has shed some light on other dietary variables that modify the caffeine effect: sugar and artificial sweeteners. Maybe the relationship between caffeine and blood pressure needs to be examined more thoroughly by taking into consideration the type and amount of sweetener. Maybe it is the sugar plus caffeine not just caffeine alone that contributes to a long-term increase of blood pressure.

Decaf for whom?

The chapter would not be complete if I leave out decaffeinated beverages. When one takes out caffeine does the remaining beverage have any effect on blood pressure? Interestingly yes and that effect is due to another substance called theobromine.

Theobromine, an alkaloid present in cacao, chocolate, tea, and coffee just like caffeine is also capable of altering blood pressure. However, theobromine action is different than that of caffeine. Theobromine does not cause blood pressure spikes. It does the opposite. Instead of narrowing blood vessels it opens them resulting in vasodilation. Theobromine is also a diuretic. It makes one pee. Because of these two properties, opening blood vessels and removing excess water, theobromine has been used successfully for lowering blood pressure.

Since regular coffee contains both caffeine and theobromine a typical brew is capable of producing two opposing heart actions. Depending on the type of coffee, its blend, brew style and preparation, coffee can produce varied effects to individuals ranging from an increase to a decrease in blood pressure. Increase due to caffeine and decrease due to theobromine. Decaffeination changes that.

But, contrary to popular belief, removing caffeine does not make coffee heart-neutral. Decaffeination removes caffeine leaving theobromine behind. Removing one substance and keeping the other makes all the difference to the cardiovascular system. Decaffeinated coffee, because of the remaining theobromine, does not increase, but actually lowers blood pressure.

Theobromine is not a stranger in medicine. *The American Journal of Clinical Nutrition* noted historic use of theobromine for arteriosclerosis, certain vascular diseases, angina pectoris, and hypertension. Thus if you have high blood pressure, pre-hypertension, white coat syndrome, morning spikes, atherosclerosis or angina say hello to decaffeinated beverages and foods that are rich in theobromine: chocolate, coffee, tea, and cacao. On the other hand, if you have low blood pressure, avoid decaf and look for beverages with high caffeine content.

Yes's and no's made easier

Uff, that was a lot of detail! Although most of it is straightforward and intuitive, you may wish to see a summary of yes's and no's in a quick-glace format, so here it is. From the blood pressure point of view

- If you have no risk for hypertension either caffeinated coffee or tea is fine;
- If you already have high blood pressure, pre-hypertension, or white coat syndrome stick to tea or decaf unless you are looking to benefit from properties of caffeine itself;
- If you have low blood pressure, decaf is not for you;
- As to pop, due to its lack of any kind of health benefits, you will be better off not drinking it regardless whether it is caffeine-free, sugar-free, or even calorie-free.

	Caffeinated coffee	*Caffeinated Tea*	*Decaf*	*Any Pop*
Normal blood pressure	*Yes*	*Yes*	*No*	*No*
Low blood pressure	*Yes + sugar*	*Yes + sugar*	*No*	*No*
High blood pressure	*Maybe, likely no*	*Maybe, likely yes*	*Yes*	*No*
Fluctuating blood pressure	*No*	*Maybe*	*Maybe*	*No*

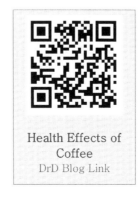

http://goo.gl/A3Pzlu

Health Effects of Coffee
DrD Blog Link

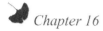 *Chapter 16*

A pinch about salt

Salt has been deemed as one of the unhealthiest condiments. It has been put next to sugar as another version of a white poison. You may have heard to stay away from it because it is really bad for you. It causes high blood pressure, heart failure, hardening or arteries, strokes, and kidney degeneration. Salt is also suspected in osteoporosis and cancer of esophagus, besides producing other nasty effects such as blood clumping and narrowing arteries.[57, 58]

I found that health-minded people are very familiar with the bad side of salt and put a real effort to reduce its intake. Some go a mile and a half not to ingest it. They investigate labels for salt content, stay away from salt-laden junk food, and would be ashamed if they own a salt shaker. But despite this enormous health effort they frequently end up with some kind of cardiovascular problem.

Overpackaged and oversalted

Salt is everywhere but the widespread use of it in food is warranted. This cheap substance can deliver flavor and at the same time preserve food for the proverbial pennies. It is thus not surprising that the food industry uses salt abundantly in their products from buns to burgers.

An average American consumes about 2 tsp. of salt a day, equivalent to 3.5g of sodium, double what's recommended. Official dietary guidelines suggest keeping sodium intake somewhere between 1.5 and 2.3 grams a day. Please understand that this is a gross simplification which neither takes into consideration an individual's health status nor blood pressure levels. Nonetheless, such one-fits-all approach is necessary to simplify matters and encourage people to lower their sodium intake.

Despite simplicity of the recommendations, the public does not follow the guidelines and there is a reason for it. There is no other way to know the salt content of the food unless one studies nutritional labels carefully. Detecting salt in food without reading labels is not an option, because one cannot rely on the taste. Even dishes tasting sweet, sour or tart may have a large amount of sodium hidden from "view."

For example, ½ cup of pasta sauce can contain 0.6g, 2 tbsp. of commercial salad dressing 0.4g, and a portion of Eggo waffles 0.6g. A portion of Raisin Bran 0.2g, 1 cup of vegetable cocktail 0.5g, 1 cup of cream-style canned corn 0.7g, canned chicken noodle soup 0.8g, 1 tbsp. of soya sauce 1g.[59]

Did you know that there is even salt in colas, fresh buns, and your favorite cheesecake? Every time you eat processed food you ingest salt. It all adds up and consumers that heavily rely on ready-made, processed and packaged goods end up with the highest sodium intake without being aware of it. Did you know that cereals and baked goods are the single largest contributor to dietary sodium intake in US and UK adults?[60]

Is everyone doomed?

Since a large chunk of the population in civilized countries rely on conveniences it is not surprising that statistically we are all overloaded with sodium. Yet, this is not true for junk-avoiding individuals, because a whopping 77% of ingested salt comes from food processing, not from home-made meals.[61]

This is how the numbers stack out. A risotto made at home has practically no sodium at all, but its commercially prepared alternative has over one gram in a portion. Similarly, homemade steak and chips usually end up with less than 0.1gram of sodium on the plate, in comparison a standard hamburger and fries has 1.3 grams.[62] That's without adding any extra salt from a salt shaker.

Salt depletion for the health conscious?

As those who eat processed foods are subject to negative effect of salt overdose, those who are health-conscientious seem to suffer the opposite— salt depletion.

Here is where low blood pressure sufferers need to perk their ears up. Do you eat mostly at home? Do you seldom use a salt shaker? Do you exercise? Are you conscious about drinking plenty of water to hydrate and detoxify? Do you talk a lot at work or home? Do you sweat when nervous? Are you prone to stress and anxiety?

If you answered yes to these questions you may have discovered the reason behind your low blood pressure: salt insufficiency.

Sodium is different from other minerals. Other minerals build bones, help in hormone production, and liver detoxification. They aid in hair growth, tooth mineralization, and skin regeneration, but sodium is not known for that. It is mostly known for its ability to expand fluids. You may have noticed this property yourself. Don't you drink gulps of water after eating at Chinese restaurants? Salt without exception makes one thirsty. It is just a matter of amount.

More salt, more water

Water follows salt and since 85% of the body's sodium is in the blood[63] it is easy to see that sodium determines blood volume. This is important from the standpoint of blood pressure, because more salt means more volume, and more volume means more pressure. The opposite is true as well: less sodium means less volume and that of course, means less pressure. Therefore, excess salt can cause hypertension, but going sodium-free can drop blood pressure in many individuals.

Salt is an essential mineral and since stress, exercise, talking, and heat cause substantial salt loss one must look into ways to replenish it. Yet, unprocessed foods and home-made dishes are typically low in salt. This is when a healthy low-sodium diet becomes problematic for low blood pressure individuals. I was unaware of this possibility until I kept a log of my salt intake. I thought I was eating healthy, but my log showed that I may be low in salt. I noticed that if I ate only home-made meals my sodium would stay at about 700 mg/day, which is a very low number. And although that covered a daily minimum of 500mg/day[64] my low-salt home-made meals could not keep my blood pressure at normal levels. I had to start consciously adding salt to up my blood pressure to feel alive.

Although there is a lot of talk about beneficial health effects of lowering sodium intake, low salt diets can be detrimental to people with low blood pressure. Low salt diets, which keep blood pressure low, may cause a lot more health problems than high salt diets in people with hypotension.

It is hard to believe, but one of the most successful treatments for hypotension is regular infusion of intravenous saline solution. A liter of normal saline (water solution containing salt) has been shown to be extremely beneficial for people with low and even fluctuating blood pressure.[65,66] But instead of finding a doctor that commits to expanding you blood vessels weekly, paying money for the service, and wasting an hour sitting in a clinic chair while being hooked up to an intravenous, you may want to employ a salt shaker instead. It is more convenient and cheaper, does not waste time, and it is definitely tastier than a plastic bag attached to your arm.

Play around with the amount of salt your body feels best with and, if your numbers are low, start a day with a well-salted blood pressure rising breakfast. Getting a salt shaker going in the morning can make a dramatic difference for the rest of the day and let you think, move, and get your life zest back.

When do I need more salt?

Don't expect that your ideal salt intake to be the same day in, day out. Because your activity level, weather, and your health status changes so do your salt needs. To know how much you need you add you need to be aware of factors that affect mineral loss. Watch out for the circumstances listed below. They are common contributors to salt loss.

- Use of **diuretics**: coffee, tea, caffeine drinks, diuretic medication, some weight loss supplements, etc.; every pee contains sodium; the more pee the more sodium loss.
- Diarrhea and **vomiting**: bodily fluids contain sodium and digestive issue can cause rapid sodium depletion; watch out especially for vomiting; stomach juices are full of sodium.
- **Heat**: heat causes shifting blood towards the skin leaving less volume for the arteries inside the body; heat also causes sweating, which depletes sodium; both can have a striking effect on blood pressure. This effect is even more pronounced in people not

accustomed to climatic changes. Studies show that people with low acclimatization have unusually high sodium loss through sweat.[67]

- **Exercise**: salt loss via sweat can be significant; intense exercise and especially if done in heat can cause substantial salt depletion.[68]
- **Physical work**: even if you don't call it exercise, physical work can cause sweating; landscaping, drain digging, construction work can make your sodium depleted and woozy in a short time, but don't forget that even light gardening in the mid-summer day can also cause a problem.
- **Diet** high in potassium and calcium, as mentioned before, can cause increased sodium excretion through urine.[69] Dairy or banana pee will be richer in sodium and there will be less sodium left to keep pressure up.
- **Stress** and anxiety: many people sweat when nervous; how much and where varies from a person to a person; the most common areas are palms, forehead, chest, armpits, or sometimes the entire body. The bigger the surface and the more sweat per square inch the more sodium is lost.
- **Infections:** do you recall getting a fever, having a rough night and waking up drenched in sweat? Sweating due to infection is not any different than sweating due to exercise, heat or stress. It all causes sodium loss.

Who can have more salt?

Most people with steady low blood pressure will greatly benefit from increased sodium intake provided they do not suffer from kidney disease. The kidneys decide on sodium concentration in urine and malfunctioning kidneys are no longer good at this task. Swollen ankles are one of the signs of water retention. Ask your doctor if your swollen ankles are preventing you from going on a higher salt diet.

People with high blood pressure may want to follow general dietary guidelines and keep their sodium low. But wait, let me rephrase it. People with high blood pressure first and foremost should avoid junk food. How they treat their salt shaker is much less important. Salt is necessary for health, but salt overload via junk food is never a good health idea.

Additionally, salt overdose may not be a problem for people with normal blood pressure, but for people with high blood pressure may not tolerate it. Those with high blood pressure not only have already expanded blood volume, but as few studies suggest, they may also react negatively to salt. So while a salty dish may make no difference for a person with normal blood pressure, people with high blood pressure can see a huge spike even after eating the same meal.

Increasing salt intake, however, is worth considering for fluctuating blood pressure. Sudden swings from extreme low to mid-high are difficult to manage with pills. Doctors have a much easier time to control a state of steady high rather than fluctuating blood pressure. Keeping blood pressure consistently a tad higher and preventing sudden otherwise unmanageable dips may be just what the body needs. Salt may turn out to be the easiest solution to erase bouts of light-headedness, fatigue, and dizziness that are due to poor circulation.

I hope by now you got over a salt phobia and are ready to infuse some energy back into the circulation. Don't think about parting with a salt shaker. If you are cleared by your doctor to do so put some generous sprinkles on your scrambled eggs, tomato, or avocado. Add that new routine to your coffee habit and you are ready to tackle the day's demands.

http://goo.gl/eB9iUU

Foods causing
High BP
DrD Blog Link

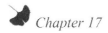 *Chapter 17*

Water works at every age

Alternative health practitioners believe that most of us are generally dehydrated. First, I thought this was a far-fetched oversimplification, but I have to attest that, as per my own clinical experience, a simple prescription of water did miracles for many patients.

Unfortunately, the proverbial eight glasses a day somehow did not get to be too popular. Many drink far less or far less for their needs. So despite a convenient access to drinking water an average North American is a bit on the dry side. The elderly lead the trend. Heat strokes, confusion, weakness, and heat fainting are common manifestation of dehydration. Better hydration could help the above, but there are many reasons why, despite negative effects of dehydration, we are shunning water.

- We are not very good at distinguishing **hunger** from thirst. And with food tasting better than plain water we end up being overfed and under-hydrated.
- Hydration sensors in the **brain** are not always working. One may not feel thirsty, yet be totally dehydrated.
- Water does not **taste** exciting; pop, beer, coffee chillers, wine are much more palatable. But these are not the same as water. These are mostly diuretics and will leave negative water balance especially if drank regularly.

- Drinking water invariably leads to more frequent **bathroom** visits. These may be inconvenient. No one wants to break a meeting, get off the bus in a rush hour, or wake up for the bathroom at the midnight hour, so we drink less to feel more comfortable.
- Leaky incontinent **bladders** are a nuisance. Some people figured that drinking less leads to less bladder rush and fewer accidents. Sneezing, coughing, and laughing may feel dryer, safer, and more comfortable in a dehydrated state.
- Permanent water **containers** do not fit in small purses and are heavy and one has to keep on carrying it even after use. They can also leak making a mess. Lighter one-time use plastic bottles are shunned as environmentally unacceptable. It takes some thinking to make water available on demand, portable, less inconvenient and less messy.
- Commercial **food** is dehydrating. Common junk snacks such as chips, pretzels, and crackers are dry and salty. So are commercially prepared lunches and dinners.
- Poor **planning**. We are so accustomed to the abundance of coffee and convenience shops that, admit it, we seldom prepare sufficiently for travel. Few think of taking water in a briefcase or car if good-tasting fresh drinks are available at any corner. But when faced with the reality of lineups and cost, we seldom respond to our thirst signals. Thus, suppressing thirst is an easy habit to develop.

Add to that the nonexistence of the almighty water-distributing Genie that would give reliable reminders, provide convenience and easier access to better-tasting water and you have a reason why a large chunk of our busy lifestyle is devoid of water.

But here is a good option for the distracted. I know of some clever phone apps that can, at least partially, replace the water Genie for you. With a jingle or a vibe they can remind you to refuel. If you are notoriously forgetful about hydration you may download the apps and have at least a mini Genie working for you.

Body checks

But what if you are already good with drinking water? How can you tell if you are still need more? Are there any checks along the way? Luckily there are.

Look at your pee. If it looks yellow, dark yellow, or orange, unless the color is from your meds, you are surely dehydrated. Still not sure? Then pinch the skin on the back of your hands and make it stand. If the fold does not flatten in one to three seconds you are lacking water.

Other signs of dehydration are more subtle and less obvious. They may range from fatigue to muscle cramps, and headaches. Chronic dehydration leads to constipation, breathing difficulties, stomach ulcers, bladder infections, loss of appetite, insomnia, palpitations, bad breath, brain fog, mood changes, weight gain, and indigestion.[70,71,72]The more serious consequences of dehydration involve seizures, brain swelling, kidney damage, and collapse.[73] Dehydration may also present as low blood and fluctuating blood pressure.

Back to salt

If you paid attention while reading the previous chapter you may remember that low blood pressure should be treated by adding extra salt to the menu. You may have already identified a salt shaker nearby, however, be aware no amount of salt will do if salt is not followed by water. If you add salt, but drink no water you will end up not only destroying your efforts to improve blood pressure, but also end up even more dehydrated.

Excess sodium must be diluted and excreted through urine or sweat, but for that you need extra water. If water is lacking sodium can accumulate (salt out) in tissues causing arterial hardening. Did you know that loss of arterial elasticity has been correlated with high salt diets?[74] Or again, let me add an already well-known detail correlated with high junk diet. Pro-inflammatory rubbish, regardless of salt intake, can turn anyone into a stiff. So eat salt, not junk, and follow up with a good amount of water to keep hydrated and flexible.

Ratios matter

You may be among a group of individuals who is absolutely convinced that you and dehydration have nothing to do with each other. After all, you drink your water diligently and your pee is pale. There is no way you are lacking water!

Dehydration is a general term for lack of water. But here is a twist. Dehydration does not refer to how little water you drink, but to insufficient amounts of water that remain in the body. You may drink three liters of water or more a day, but if that water gets peed out instead of reaching your tissues your organs will still be dehydrated. This is where salt comes in.

Salt and water are like a brother and sister. In the body they go together, but they must stay in the right proportion. Your body needs 1 part sodium for approximately 100 parts of water. Normal saline, an intravenous bag of salty water given in hospitals contains exactly of 0.9% sodium, the most hydrating water to salt ratio.

Because good hydration requires this specific ratio it is incorrect to think that dehydration originates solely from poor water drinking habits. Dehydration can also stem from maintaining wrong water to salt proportions. When you think about it for a moment you may figure out that there is not just one type of dehydration, but two—one due to excess sodium and insufficient water and the other to insufficient water, which is due to insufficiency of salt. The earlier is more common in hypertension. The latter dominates low and fluctuating blood pressure.

Healthy with low blood pressure?

Without sufficient salt water cannot stay in tissues. The body will dispose of it, even though it needs it. Many healthy folks report that water "goes through them" as soon as it is drank. It is hard to believe, but despite drinking liters of water one can still stay dehydrated.

I met a lot of health-conscious folks only to find out they suffered from low blood pressure, brain fog, fatigue, and lack of zest. I also found out that these were people who avoided salt thinking that it is bad, maniacally exercised thinking that it is good, and at the same time drank lots of plain water thinking that is a necessary prescription for health. Invariably, they were puzzled as to why, despite putting so much effort into being healthy, they didn`t feel good.

If drinking gallons of water does not guarantee hydration should you continue upping your water intake or should you take more salt? Things can get complicated, so to prevent confusion I made a simple summary for you. With this handy guide you can start hydrating better today.

	Urine - darker	*Urine - watery*
Normal blood pressure	*More water*	*Less water*
Low and fluctuating blood pressure	*Definitely more water*	*More salt*
High blood pressure	*Definitely more water*	*Check kidneys*

Too much water is not good either

Since we are on the topic of hydration I cannot omit talking about over-hydration. Over-hydration is nothing else but excess water in the body, regardless of the salt intake. Symptoms of over-hydration may be too few and too vague to notice. Among them are: confusion, headaches, lethargy, and distractibility.[75] If you have any of the above and your pee is pale cut down on water and see if things change. Don't overhydrate. As much as we need water on a daily basis, too much of it can actually kill you.

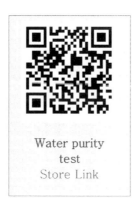

Water purity
test
Store Link

http://goo.gl/VKgLhr

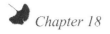 *Chapter 18*

Are you nuts about coconuts?

Coconut water has been used as a standard hydrating beverage in many tropical countries, but its popularity in North America is relatively recent. Coconut water has been marketed, not without a reason, as a health-promoting beverage.

Coconut water has significant anti-ageing, anti-carcinogenic, and anti-stroke effects.[76] It is also a powerful antioxidant due to a dense arrangement of inorganic ions. Besides being rich in calcium, magnesium, and sodium it is extremely rich in potassium. Just one cup of coconut water has over 600mg of this mineral,[77] definitely more than a well-known potassium king, banana.

Exactly due to its mineral density and a heart-friendly ratio of sodium to potassium coconut water is exceptionally useful for hypotension. Coconut water expands blood volume, which in turn increases blood pressure. One to two cups a day may be enough to make a day zestful, lively, and strong instead of weak, fatigued, and dull.

Coconut water is excellent at times when one gets "stranded" without food and has no access to snacks, coffee, or other blood pressure boosters. Coconut water is rich in nutrients and has enough sugars and salts to bring a person from low to high without giving jitters, which is not uncommon with sugary snacks or coffee overdose.

Feel free to experiment with coconut water unless your doctor told you that you have kidney or adrenal problems, diabetic acidosis or heart disease. If you easily accumulate potassium in the blood get medical clearance before eating bananas or drink coconut water.

Did you know that coconut water is so blood-similar that in case of emergency it could be used directly as an intravenous hydrating drip?[78] Filtered coconut water has been used as an intravenous plasma alternative successfully in many countries including Cuba, Honduras, Sri Lanka, Japan, and Solomon Islands.[79] But regardless how exciting it may sound, please refrain from intravenous experimentations. It won't go well. To enjoy coconut water safely limit it to oral intake.

Beware of differences

Before you head out to stack your kitchen pantry with coconut water ensure you are getting the real thing. If you haven't gotten into a habit of reading labels yet the time is now. Although it may feel tedious, annoying, and bothersome, know that reading labels is as important as having a poop in the morning. If you don't do it, sooner or later you end up in trouble.

So turn that bottle or can around and rest your eyes on a line that says "ingredients." This is important. Even though the front says "coconut water" you may be surprised what else is inside. Unless the ingredient list has only one item listed: coconut water, put it back on a store shelf. If you want results you need to get the real and unprocessed variety. Everything else may end up in disappointment.

Also do not confuse coconut water with coconut milk. They are two totally different products. The first one is a watery liquid (94% water), the other a white thick substance (only 50% water).[80] Coconut milk would not be helpful to raise blood pressure. In fact over time it can do the opposite.[81]

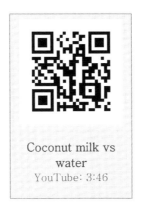

Coconut milk vs
water
YouTube: 3:46

https://youtu.be/IWvdn_5nfHs

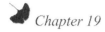 *Chapter 19*

The best time to exercise is...

Have you noticed that there is a special time of the day when you feel your best? It may be right after rising, late afternoon, after coffee or a cold shower. Maybe you haven't given it much though, but is it possible that these energy peaks and valleys have anything to do with blood pressure?

Blood pressure, as you know from previous chapters, fluctuates. It goes low at night and stays high in the day, but it not only does that. Blood pressure changes significantly also during the day-time hours. There are specific times of the day when blood pressure stays low and times of the day when blood pressure stays high.

People with normal blood pressure may not care about the circadian rhythms of circulation, but people with low or fluctuating blood pressure should take notice, because an increase or decrease of mere few points may translate to a noticeable change in energy. Smart and health-conscious people will benefit by reorganizing details of the day to fit biological laws and take advantage of lows and highs of the heart.

Time yourself well

Mental, physical, and emotional capacity also varies throughout the day. Ten a.m. is known as the time of alertness peak.[82] Ten a.m. is the best time for mental activities such as learning, reading, writing, and communicating. At that time you may write your best essay on improving relationships or come up with an innovative solution to world garbage problems, but you most likely won't break the world record in sprint or javelin. Ten a.m. is not the time for performing the most stunning physical feats, especially if your blood pressure keeps staying low.

You may think the best time to exercise is in the morning, but what do you do if the body says you are "not up to it?" Should you force yourself into a cardiovascular effort that may not be even paying off? In that case it may be to your advantage to listen to your body and shift your fitness routine to the p.m. Your body may be readier for physical stunts in the afternoon, because the highest cardiovascular efficiency and muscle strength is known to be around 5 p.m.[83] Interestingly, this physical peak falls exactly at the time of the highest blood pressure.

That's not to say that everyone should exercise in the afternoon, but people with low blood pressure may want to take advantage of this double gain in p.m. hours: stronger muscles and harder pumping heart. However, if your high blood pressure is a tad on a high side don't shift your fitness routine yet. Instead, consider staying away from weight lifting in the late afternoon unless you have blood pressure under control. A hypertensive heart does not need any more stress at 5 p.m.

Avoid the surges

If your blood pressure is not always low or always high, but does funny things, spikes and dips at unpredictable moments, then you may want to put a thought about morning exercise away for good. Although the highest blood pressure is typically recorded between 3 p.m. and 9 p.m., the highest *surge* in blood pressure is around 7 a.m. This is when blood pressure shows the sharpest rise upwards within 24-hour cycle.[84]

This increase is not without consequences. Acute cardiovascular episodes such as heart attacks and strokes are most common at that time.[85] The highest cardiovascular mortality is in the morning hours, exactly the hours that record the sharpest rise in blood pressure. If your blood pressure is erratic make sure to tell your doctor to adjust the meds and stay away from lifting heavy objects upon rising.

Lifting weights is known to challenge the cardiovascular system the most. Lifting increases blood pressure higher than any other activity, but this effect is only during the time of the actual act of lifting, called active lift, not in between or afterwards.[86] So while you are lifting blood pressure surges upwards, once you put the weights down blood pressure takes a nosedive. This is why some get a broken vessel and some feel dizzy or faint during a weight lifting session.

Since this blood pressure ups and downs do not apply only to dumbbells be aware of this cardiovascular capriciousness with every item or grocery bag you handle. Observe and teach yourself to stay within your exertion limits. If you experience dizziness with exercise, don't stop your physical activities. Just lower the weight and increase the reps.

Don't hold your breath!

If weight lifting is your thing, but the blood pressure surges uncontrollably there is a way to calm the heart without you having to give up the gym.

Despite the fact that weight lifting, especially leg presses, cause an incredible blood pressure surge, not uncommonly higher than 300/200mmHg, don't back down from the gym yet! Studies done on weight lifters demonstrated that blood pressure can be modified depending what you do with the breath. Breath holding while pressing or pushing increases blood pressure. Breathing out while lifting prevents those nasty surges.

One study measured blood pressure on athletes during exercises. The participants were asked to do simple leg presses in two different ways. One way was to press while holding breath, the other way was to do leg presses while doing slow exhalation. The differences turn out to be significant.

The average athletes' blood pressure during presses with breath holding was 311/284mmHg (!), but while doing slow exhalation it was only 198/175mmHg. That's an incredible difference worth paying attention to, because regardless of what your cardiovascular surge is, to prevent strokes and burst blood vessels you need to think how you breathe. Never hold your breath while lifting, pushing, or pressing. Exercise is much safer that way.[87]

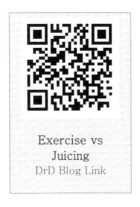

Exercise vs
Juicing
DrD Blog Link

http://goo.gl/hCIL7q

More Symptoms

Tests & Tips

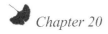 *Chapter 20*

Morning allergies that are not

Anxiety, ringing in ears, kidney malfunction, memory problems and glaucoma are all well-studied effects of decreased blood flow, but can a runny nose fit in that equation? There haven't been gobs of studies on the subject, yet my clinical experience indicates that many hypotensives not only end up waking up groggy, but also on the verge of a cold. Runny nose, chilliness, and a slight soreness of throat is not uncommon among those with low blood pressure.

The morning sniffles do not usually extend to the later part of the day although they are seldom replaced by a feeling of robustness. Since the "cold" neither persists nor develops into a full-blown infection it is seldom mentioned to anyone. One just "lives with it."

Morning ill health may repeat day in and day out somehow improving during summer months and worsening during winter. Many get accustomed to the "morning allergies" and do not think much about them. However, a sensation that something is wrong with the immune system and a persistent feeling of coldness usually does not go away. Interestingly, as per my observations, that recurrent morning pattern does not seem to extend to people with high blood pressure.

Beyond the obvious

Nothing in the body happens by chance, not even that morning runny nose. Everything is connected and runs via extensive feedback loops. A knee scrape will be registered simultaneously by the skin, hormonal, immune, and circulatory systems. These systems will all act to seal the skin, prevent infection, improve blood flow to the area, and repair the wound. If the knee scrape does not want to go away one needs to look beyond the cuts and connect "why" dots. Maybe the immune system cannot handle the laceration or maybe the circulatory system does not bring enough blood to the area. The nose is not any different than the knee. If the nose keeps on running there is a reason for it.

Low blood pressure is invariably related to lower perfusion, "slower" circulation and consequently colder body temperature. That's why people with low blood pressure get colder easier and are more prone to cold hands and feet. This chilling effect has further undesirable ramifications, including developing virus-friendly body milieu.

Welcome to the land of rhinovirus

The most common cold virus is called rhinovirus. Not that it makes any difference to you, however, it is sometimes good to know what's "bugging" you. The most important thing about this cold virus is that it likes to keep cold. The virus gets the most amorous and makes babies in a hurry at 33-35°C (91-95 °F), which is 1-2 degrees Celsius below normal body temperature. It is not difficult to see that if your body stays in a sub-normal temperature zone you may end up as a cold virus host.

Core temperature changes throughout the day. It is usually the lowest at night and in the morning when you move the least.[88] But even if the room is cold, and sheets are thin, the body temperature should keep at the healthy level. A runny nose may just mean that your body temperature is lower than it should be. Pull a thermometer out, test yourself, and put an end to those mysterious "allergies."

BBT test

The test to measure your morning core temperature is called BBT. BBT is an abbreviation for a basal body temperature, a test that measures overall metabolic robustness. You want to do this test because besides immune system it can also help you with weight loss. Low BBT means slow metabolism and this means you will have a hard time losing weight unless you seriously under eat.

You will do this test first thing in the morning while still in bed, so ensure that a working thermometer is within your reach. To be on the safe side put it on your night table the night before.

When you wake up do not go anywhere. Don't uncover, go to the bathroom, sip water, or scratch your itch. Stay still. Slowly reach for your thermometer. Keep in bed under covers and relax. Wait until the measurement is done and then compare your temperature. Normal oral temperature should be around 36.6°C (97.9°F).

Lower temperatures such as oral temperature below 36.3°C (97.3°F) may be contributing to viral replication and recurring colds. Do not be surprised if you see 34.5°C (94.1°F) or 35.5°C (95.9°F) on your thermometer. Such low temperatures *are* common in low metabolic and low immune system states. If you have low blood pressure, low BBT and recurring colds you must boost your blood pressure and body temperature before your nose stops sniffling.

Take a good look at your leaky nose. Are you still spraying it to make it dryer? Now think for a moment. If your "morning allergies" are due to low immune system, low temperature, and poor blood flow does it make any sense to use sprays to dry your nose? They neither boost immunity, increase temperature, or contribute to better circulation.

Here is healthy financial advice: don't spend endless money on popular Dristans, Sudafeds or any other nose-drying spray. You will only throw your money away in exchange for a few hours of relief. Instead, look into permanent health-building solution. Health is a skill, not a pill, potion, injection, or a cream. And for sure health does not come conveniently packed as a nose spray.

Warming Foods
Chart
Download

http://goo.gl/87XTCD

Cooling Foods
Chart
Download

http://goo.gl/OFKNku

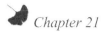 *Chapter 21*

Immune boosting at home

Believe it or not, but there are ways to boost the immune system, and you don't need to give your soul away to the devil, or a Mexican clinic for that matter. You don't need a team of specialist looking over your shoulders twenty-four hours a day, sophisticated hi-tech gadgets, intravenous hookups, or a line-up of newly discovered pharmaceuticals, because the simplest and the most practical method to boost the immune system does not require any of that.

You may also be surprised that you don't need a referral or any prescription from your medical doctor. Conventional medicine is thin when it comes to building health. Just realize that pharmacy shelves are full of immuno-suppressive drugs, but slim on immuno-boosting pills. Immune system building is not a field conventional medicine excels in, so don't waste your time on standard prescriptions. Science is yet to discover a pill for health, robustness, and a strong immune system. Health building is a skill and a "do it yourself" project, not a capsule or an implant.

Natural medicine is on your side

You may be luckier while peeking onto shelves of a health food store. Natural medicine has many excellent aids for the immune system. You are probably familiar with well-researched vitamin C and vitamin D, both of which are used successfully even in the most immune-compromised cases, including cancer or AIDS. The fame of these immune-boosting vitamins has infiltrated conventional medicine over time. Nowadays these vitamins are used as main or supportive therapies in the most progressive conventional clinics, but the progress towards understanding how to build health is slow. Sadly, you still can find doctors that up to this day "don't believe in vitamins."

Herbs also have immuno-boosting properties. Adaptogens such as astragalus, ginger, panax, among other herbs have been shown to help build immune strength over time. In fact, just walk in to a health food isle and you will be surprised how many bottles line up to help you overcome colds, flus, allergies, bee stings, hives, fatigue, and poor stamina. But remember pills are pills. Once you start with them you need to continue, because they only work when you take them.

Water wonders

For those who do not want to be married to pills and got chained to the ongoing financial drain there is a great immuno-building and blood pressure-regulating solution all in one. It is called hydrotherapy.

Hydrotherapy is a fancier term for use of water for healing purposes. Water is not only a foundation of life, but it is well-known prescription among healing arts enthusiasts. Modern hygiene uses water for washing and rinsing to get rid of dirt and germs. Clean water is the simplest cleaning solvent known and hand washing prevents infections. But properties of water go further than that. Water can be used to boost both the immune as well as cardiovascular system.

Hydro-works

Hydrotherapy abounds in health-promoting practices. From vaginal douches to sitz baths to steam saunas hydrotherapy has wide applications from shrinking hemorrhoids to skin rejuvenation. This incredible versatility of water is due to its specific physical properties, mainly its ability to change temperature and pressure.

Healing with water is nothing new. The practices were recorded by ancient Egyptians, Romans, Persian, and Greek civilizations.[89] Both royalties and public enjoyed water's healing properties. Today hydrotherapy is used by naturopaths, occupational therapists, physiotherapists, and has evolved into sophisticated medical treatments including rehab pools for dogs and cryotherapy in sports medicine.

Despite technical advancement and updated scientific insight, water healing properties did not change. You can still use water in the comfort of your home for multiple health benefits. It will work the same way as it did in the ancient Roman empire pleasing royalties as well as today's sophisticated spas enthralling celebrities.

Immuno-building with water

Immuno-building with water is extremely simple. You do not need any machinery, essential oils, perfumes, lotions, potions, flower petals, or highly advertised and coincidently highly expensive "must have" health toys. In fact, hydrotherapy is the cheapest and the most convenient immune system boost you can receive. It is such a simple "do it yourself" technique that eliminates the need for doctors, technicians, spouses, or servants.

Starting today you can turn your bathroom into a modern health facility without costly renovations or hiring specialized teams. You can harness immune and cardiovascular benefits of water at whim. So if you think your health needs repairing, stop coming up with yet another excuse and delay. Part the shower curtain and step into better health.

Hot and cold, or just cold

Add immune-boosting power to your shower by changing water temperature in the following way. Start with your typical shower. The water may be warm, hot, or tepid depending on your liking. Don't change that. Continue your normal shower routine as usual and reserve your one-minute daily immune-boost to the very end.

This is when instead of turning the tap off and stepping out of the shower, you are turning off hot water only. Leave cold water running and stay inside the shower despite an irresistible urge to run away. This chilling moment is not to your detriment. This is exactly when health building happens, so stick with it. Less adventurous individuals can turn off hot water partially, so the water is semi-cold, not chilling-cold. This modification is a good beginning, but it is not as effective as super cold soak.

Don't cringe! It's worth it!

Studies are very clear that temperature altering hydrotherapy does have an incredible effect on our bodies. Cold invigorates and stimulates. Warmth releases tension and relaxes. Sudden temperature change redirects blood flow, challenges metabolism, and activates detoxification.[90]

A cold shower is not only invigorating, but also changes many vital immune system parameters. Repeated cold water stimulations reduce frequency of infections, increases white blood cell counts, and regulate inflammatory responses. Daily brief cold water stress has been shown to enhance anti-tumor immunity, and boost antiviral and anti-cancer factors.[91] Brief cold hydrotherapy is quickly becoming a novel therapy for weakened and immunocompromised, including cancer and AIDS patients.

Cold-water immersion increases metabolic rate and stabilizes core temperature, exactly what you need if your BBT test turned out imperfect. Did you know that just one hour bath in 20°C (68°F) nearly doubles metabolic rate of the body and lower temperature increase it even more? One hour bath at 14°C (57°F) boosts the metabolic rate by a whopping 350%! Remember, colder is better, at least when it comes to raising body temperature.[92] And no, you do not have to turn a cold bathtub into your permanent residence to increase body temperature and accelerate weight loss. Even quick cold showers, when done daily, can do that for you.

Love your brown fat!

Cold helps build brown fat. Don't panic! Brown fat is not the same jiggly bulge around your navel you want to get rid of. It is the type of fat you actually want. This type of fat, abundant in newborns, keeps the body temperature up. Unfortunately, over time brown fat is replaced by less metabolically active and less burnable white adipose tissue, the spare tire you are well familiar with.[93]

Loss of brown fat is not good for the body. Lack of it leads to temperature sensitivity, lower metabolic rate, poorer immunity, and obesity. Since white coat syndrome and hypertension is more common in overweight people,[94] cold showers may just be the right thing to do. Studies show that exposure to extreme cold can produce a fifteen-fold increase in brown fat which can result in a nine-pound weight loss over a year.[95] And that's without changing the diet!

Here is a little bit of a road block for people on high blood pressure medication. Beta-blockers, a type of popular anti-hypertensive drug, can cause brown fat disappearance.[96] And loss of brown fat has known consequences ranging from weight gain to inability to deal with temperature changes. Ever wondering why you are getting colder, fatter, and sicker? Check your blood pressure meds and focus on getting your brown fat back.

Choose your temperature wisely

You have to be patient with brown fat. It does not grow overnight. It takes weeks or months to cultivate it, but don`t despair. Hydrotherapy does not only have long-term effects. It can produce significant changes in circulation right away. It can lower or raise blood pressure immediately depending on water temperature. The general rule is: cold water stimulates and hot water inhibits blood flow. To increase heart rate and blood pressure you need a cold bath. A hot bath will slow circulation down and do the opposite.

One hour cold bath at 14°C (57°F) has been shown to cause an 8% increase in blood pressure and a 5% increase in heart rate. To compare, one hour extra warm bath at 32°C (90°F) water lowers blood pressure by 12%.[97] Keep that in mind when taking baths. Avoid warm or extra warm baths if you have low or fluctuating blood pressure. Warm water will only contribute to you feeling lethargic and dizzy.

Without showers or baths

Even though you may not be tempted by and keep staying away from cold showers you can still use water to benefit circulation. Mere drinking water may be sufficient in some cases. Did you know that drinking cold water, not unlike cold baths and showers, also increases blood pressure? Studies show that two glasses of cold water can increase blood pressure by an average 33mmHg systolic and 16mmHg diastolic 30 min after ingestion.[98]

Although young and healthy individuals may not see much effect, older individuals and people with compromised circulation will definitely notice it.[99] The drinking cold water trick can help people get back on their feet and clear up foggy brains. It can also help the elderly avoid falls and prevent blood-donor fainting after donation.

Interestingly, water blood pressure rising effect is not due to blood volume expansion, but by stimulation of the nervous system, the same way coffee and cigarettes do. If so, is it then possible to switch from espresso and smokes to plain water and get the same kick? Although one may think it is impossible the studies disagree. Two cups of cold water effect on nervous system is equivalent to smoking two unfiltered cigarettes or drinking 2.5 cups of caffeinated coffee.[100] Amazing!

Foods that boost
immune system
Download

http://goo.gl/uELW4K

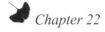 *Chapter 22*

Ortho... what?

Mornings can be challenging for people with low blood pressure. Blood pressure dipping at night, low cortisol in the morning, overnight dehydration, low salt diet, water-flushing effect of alcohol and coffee from the day before all contribute to lethargic mornings.

If you wake up with...

- Sleepiness, fatigue despite sleeping well
- Weakness, faintness even when in bed
- Confusion, light-headedness without any head trauma
- Coldness, chilliness even under covers
- Morning cold, and allergy-like symptoms
- Nausea, lack of appetite

... chances are your blood pressure ended up in a basement

Sluggish morning, sluggish day

Fortunately for many folks that morning sluggishness disappears once they move about, hydrate, eat something salty, drink coffee and keep away from alcohol, but there is a group of folks who may feel light-headed, exhausted, and weak past the morning.

For those the feeling of yuck may continue for the rest of the day, getting worse with exertion or any sudden movement. The less fortunate may end up with nausea and even lose appetite, but skipping meals will only make matters worse. It will further lower blood pressure contributing to weakness and confusion. Confusion is the enemy of making health-smart decisions. Once at that point a vicious cycle of ill-health starts perpetuating.

The above paragraph describes a reality for many seniors today: feeling worse with exertion and not any better after eating. If you or your parents belong to that category you need to get familiar with the concept of "orthostatic hypotension."

Ortho… what?

Don't be scared by that fancy name. Medical language may sound intimidating, but remember it was invented by people for people and anyone can understand it. "Orthostatic hypotension" is not any different. "Orthostatic" translated into plain English means "standing up." "Hypotension" refers to low blood pressure. So "orthostatic hypotension" simply means a drop of blood pressure upon standing up.

Because it involves changes in the posture "orthostatic hypotension" is also called "postural hypotension." Postural hypotension is not uncommon and it causes a big health concern for patients and doctors alike.

Getting to know ortho… what

Have you ever gotten up from sitting to suddenly black out or get dizzy? Have you risen up from bending to see the world spinning? Have you lost your balance after climbing a few stairs or doing squats in a gym? If yes, you may have personally experienced episodes of postural hypotension. Postural hypotension is seldom recognised or diagnosed, but causes a real challenge to many people.

Orthostatic hypotension is not a new disease. In fact, it is not a disease at all. It is well known to health practitioners as a cardiovascular anomaly. But despite its long-standing recognition, the consensus on its clear-cut definition came rather recently in 2011.[101]

Today the name "orthostatic hypotension" does not apply to any minor drop of blood pressure on standing, but has specific diagnostic criteria. The drop needs to be significant in the magnitude of at least 20 mmHg systolic or 10 mmHg diastolic.[102]

But don't get me wrong. Lesser drops of blood pressure do exist and do cause concern. Nonetheless, from a technical point of view they cannot be called orthostatic hypotension. Remember that when you want to discuss this topic with a medical doctor.

 Despite the many troubles caused by orthostatic hypotension, it is commonly overlooked. Very few clinicians routinely test for postural blood pressure changes and orthostatic symptoms may elude any patient. Although some people complain of blurred vision, headache, neck ache, palpitations, sweating, nausea, or experience a fall, not everyone has the foresight to link these symptoms to blood pressure. What makes things more complicated is the fact that not everyone has to experience those symptoms. Some people may not have any of the above at all except chronic fatigue that comes from nowhere and does not want to go away.[103]

Orthostatic hypotension is not part of a routine physical, so chances are you have never been tested for it. Good news is that the test is simple enough for you to do at home. All you need to have is a blood pressure monitor. Even though you may be compelled to think that orthostatic hypotension does not apply to you, I would like you to test anyhow. You never know.

One in three has it

Postural hypotension is very common and it tends to increase with age. As only 5% of the healthy young population will have a noticeable blood pressure drop on standing,[104] about 68% institutionalized elderly live with it.[105]

Prescription medications make things worse. Studies show that blood pressure drops affects only one in three elderly that live medication free, but twice that many if they are on meds. Two thirds of seniors who are on three prescription drugs have unstable blood pressure.[106] Not all drugs contribute to fluctuating blood pressure, but there are few that are most responsible for the orthostatic drop. These are: *antihypertensives* such as Terazosin, Hydrtochlorothiazide and Lisinopril, *diuretics* such as Furosamide, and an *antidepressants* Trazodone.[107]Check your medicine cabinet.

Orthostatic hypotension seems to also plague people suffering from certain diseases. Diabetes and Parkinson's disease aggravate blood pressure fluctuations the most. Half of all people diagnosed with Parkinson`s disease are also diagnosed with orthostatic hypotension.[108] Orthostatic hypotension not only causes poorer quality of life, increases life restrictions, but is associated with higher chances of death. Orthostatic hypotension contributes to fainting and falling,[109] and is also linked to heart failure, arrhythmia, and cognitive decline.[110] Orthostatic *incidents* are not reserved to seniors only. Apparently, nearly every third "healthy" individual experiences it.[111] So healthy or not, pull out your blood pressure cuff and get ready for testing.

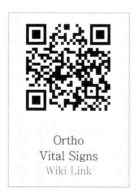

Ortho
Vital Signs
Wiki Link

https://goo.gl/P62gzC

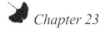 *Chapter 23*

Ortho test details

The orthostatic test is simple, but needs to be done properly to eliminate errors. You can do the test by yourself, but it would be best if there is somebody with you during the test. She/he can help you keep track of time, write down the numbers, and also assist in case you feel faint.

Preparation

1. Ensure your blood pressure monitor is in working order. Check the batteries.
2. Find a sofa/bed/bench you can comfortably lie down on. If you are prone to seeing stars or feel dizzy on standing keep close to a wall or something you may hold on to during the test.
3. Put a blood pressure cuff on your left arm and lie down.

Actual test

4. **Lie down**: Stay motionless after lying down for about a minute to let blood pressure come down to its resting state.
5. **Test BP**: Start the blood pressure monitor and have somebody record the reading. Write down all the three numbers, not just two. The third number will be useful for a different test later. In the meantime, don't get up or move or the test will be invalid. Do not take your cuff off as yet.

6. **Stand up:** Stand up quickly. Do not sit up, but stand up on your feet.

7. **Test BP:** Immediately re-start your blood pressure monitor. Keep your left arm straight. Any bending or arm jerking may invalidate the readings. Have somebody record the results, all three numbers.

8. **Keep standing for three minutes:** Keep on standing motionlessly. If you feel unbearably lightheaded you will need to stop the test and lie down to prevent fainting. Otherwise keep standing for three minutes.

9. **Test BP:** Retest your blood pressure at the end of three minutes. Record all three numbers.

Assessment

1. Did your systolic (**top number**) dropped by **20 points** from the initial reading at any time during the test?

2. Did your diastolic (**bottom number**) dropped by **10 points** from the initial reading at any time during the test?

If you have answered yes to any of these two questions you have experienced orthostatic hypotension.

To ensure that your assessment is reliable repeat the ortho test on different occasions. Check yourself on a day when you feel fatigued, when your blood pressure is low, after a stressful week, when the weather is rainy, and days when blood pressure is good.

Testing at different times can be very telling. You can learn whether your blood pressure drops constantly or is dependent on various circumstances like weather, stress, fatigue, hunger, etc. Orthostatic hypotension that happens constantly is much harder to control and may require medical intervention. Occasional orthostatic events are much easier to deal with and you may be able to control them yourself.

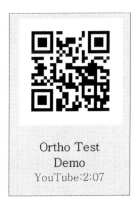

Ortho Test
Demo
YouTube:2:07

https://youtu.be/d7MVuwhiqwE

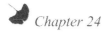 *Chapter 24*

Ortho test analysis

If you've done the test and got the results you likely want to know what they mean. There are five categories your blood pressure could have fallen into. These are:

1. BP **went up**. That`s good. You will learn in details what it means in Chapter 29.
2. BP **went down**, but no not enough for a diagnosis of orthostatic hypotension. Your adrenals may need support. Read Chapter 29 and 30.
3. BP went down beyond the diagnostic point of **orthostatic hypotension**. Oops! Treatment required. Keep on reading.
4. BP did not go down or up, but you felt **worse after the test**. You may have delayed orthostatic hypotension. Chapter 26 is for you.
5. BP did not make a large shift, but you felt your **heart racing**. You may have "orthostatic tachycardia." It will be explained in Chapter 32.

If your blood pressure went up, that`s generally a good sign, but if the blood pressure went down or you felt worse later you should now look at your notes to check *when* the blood drop occurred.

There are three distinctive patterns of falling blood pressure.[112] They have different timings, slightly different symptoms, different causes, and happen to different age groups. They also present a different level of concern. Some are non-concerning at all, and some accompany serious degenerative changes. The least concerning drops are the one that happen right away after standing.

Drop within thirty seconds

Short-lasting blood pressure shifts that occur within 30 seconds upon standing are the least alarming. They are most likely to happen in younger individuals. They may lead to temporary dizziness, but rarely to fainting. If you fall in this category, take precaution, but do not worry too much. Immediate blood pressure dips do not signify a big health problem and are easily rectified.

Drop within three minutes

Blood pressure dips that happen after thirty seconds but still fall within the first three minutes are more concerning than the previously described type. This kind of cardiovascular behavior is associated with palpitations, hearing and visual disturbances, sweating, or heart pain. This semi-delayed blood pressure drop is frequently aggravated by diuretics and cardiac drugs, but it may also be a sign of a more serious pathology.

Drop after thirty minutes

If a dip in blood pressure does not occur within three minutes, but is very delayed, possibly even by forty-five minutes, the situation is very serious. It usually accompanies very poor health and may even signify an autonomic nervous system failure. Watch out for sweating, back pain, and weakness which can happen before the person collapses. Older individuals are the most affected.

Tips for dropping blood pressure

If your test results fall into any of the three described above scenarios get familiar with the tips below. They will help you avoid sudden dizziness and even prevent falls. They do not repair underlying faulty physiology, but at least they help preventing sudden blood pressure dips.

- **Drink water**. Get into a habit of drinking water frequently, especially when you talk a lot or sweat a lot. Talking and sweating contribute to water loss. Dehydration contributes to fainting; drinking rehydrates and cold water increases blood pressure.[113]

- **Move about**. Moving the legs improves circulation and prevents blood pooling; stay away from long car rides and avoid prolonged standing. If you have to, remember to balance it with exercises. Contract the muscles below the waist for thirty seconds at a time. Alternate toe lifting, with bending at the waist, rising legs, or contracting thighs. These exercises help maintain blood pressure.[114]

- **Keep cool**. Heat makes low blood pressure worse; avoid crowded and heated places; stay inside air-conditioning malls rather than lying on scorching beaches.

- **Don't panic**. Emotional distress, especially fear is a major contributing factor to fainting.

- **Sit down**. Sit down while yawning, coughing, sneezing, eating, and peeing. These activities can slow down the heart rate, which can be followed by a sudden blood pressure drop.

- **Avoid blowing**. Sit down while playing a brass instrument; just like sneezing and yawning, blowing and breath holding slows down heart rate; even better, switch to playing a guitar.

- **Stay away from heavy objects**. Be vigilant during and after exercise; vigorous full body movements are very demanding on cardiovascular system; weightlifting is especially challenging; don't unless you are sure about your blood pressure whereabouts.

- **Steady your neck**. Skip neck exercises altogether; certain neck movements and neck rubbing can significantly lower blood pressure; leave your neck alone
- **Avoid neck rubs**. Tell your massage therapist about your condition; neck contains blood pressure regulators and rubbing or massaging them will slow down the heart and produce significant low blood pressure symptoms; stick to invigorating massages below the neck only.
- **Shrink varicose veins**. Take care of varicose veins; they can cause blood pooling and prevent blood pressure spikes when your body needs them; shrink them, or use stockings for a temporary relief.

Keep these simple common sense precautions in mind. Pass them on to your parents or older individuals, because unfit or frail people are most vulnerable to fluctuating blood pressure and its consequences. Although the tips can be used with good results I would want to encourage anyone with unstable blood pressure to put more emphasis on cardiovascular fitness as a more permanent solution.

Tips for
fluctuating BP
Download

http://goo.gl/12mBEj

Chapter 25

A dangerous act of peeing

If you think that falls happen only during the day and lying in bed is the safest time you are far from the truth. It is exactly the night that presents unexpected health risks. A combination of a finicky bladder and unpredictable whereabouts of the blood pressure at night may be sure a prescription for a nighttime disaster.

Have you heard of people fainting in a bathroom? These are not old wives' tales. Bathroom fainting is a well-documented fact. And it is not as uncommon as you may think. About one in ten people faint at least once in their lifetime during urination?[115] But why people tumble down at the toilet is no longer a mystery. We don't have to blame thick bathroom darkness and a non-existing soap on the floor for the falls any longer. Science has a much better explanation.

Just as yawning, coughing, sneezing, and eating, peeing also causes a temporary blood pressure lowering effect. Not surprisingly nighttime low blood pressure, sudden rising, and the act of peeing may all be too much for a cardiovascular system. The combination of these three factors can lead to fainting in susceptible individuals.

Fainting numbers

It takes quite a drop in blood pressure to cause loss of consciousness. Fainting does not happen with any random blood pressure drop. Even though one may feel tired, groggy and lifeless with 100/50 mmHg, this won't be enough for a black out. Fainting happens only when blood pressure reaches exceptionally low number. Usually it has to be below 60mmHg.[116] Pay attention, as this number does not pertain to the diastolic (bottom) number, but to the systolic (top) reading. Consequently blood pressure of 100/50 mmHg won't make a person collapse, but 50/30 mmHg definitely will.

Micturition syncope AKA fainting from bathroom trips at night happens, not surprisingly, to older individuals as both blood pressure and bladder control gets more unpredictable with age. It also is more common in males, as their urination-assisting projectile members operate best on standing. The faintings are not without consequences. Thirty per cent end up with cuts and bruises, but twelve per cent may break a bone.[117]

Prevention is the key

Accidents are accidents. They are never preplanned, so when you find yourself dizzy on getting up at night or in the morning take precautions. Although stopping bladder from waking you up may not be an option there are a few things you can do the night before to prevent sudden falls.

- **Drink water**. Drink enough water during the day to prevent dehydration; dehydration contributes to low blood pressure.
- **Avoid alcohol.** Avoid drinking alcohol at night; alcohol is dehydrating.
- **Eat.** Do not go to bed hungry; eat something before retiring; low blood sugar can contribute to blood pressure drop.
- **Use salt.** Do not avoid salt; it can keep your blood pressure higher.

- **Engage your MD.** Ask your doctor to switch the timing of your blood pressure medication (if you use them) to prevent overly pronounced drop of blood pressure at night.
- **Cool your bedroom.** Keep your bedroom cooler; heat causes sweating, which can contribute to dehydration.
- **Pee before bed.** Urinate before going to bed; this may prevent you from having to rush to the bathroom in the middle of the night when the blood pressure is the lowest.
- **Compress veins.** Wear compression socks to bed especially if you have varicose veins; compression socks will prevent blood from pooling in the legs.
- **Use spices.** Add cayenne powder to your socks at night; this trick improves circulation.
- **Consider wet sock therapy.** For long-term improvement of circulation in the legs consider wet socks, a grandma therapy for poor circulation.

Also:

- **Go slow.** If you have to go at night sit down in bed first and then lean forward; stay like that for a minute and then get up slowly; this maneuver prevents rapid blood pressure drops.
- **Go easy.** Do not strain while on a toilet; straining activates the vagus nerve that slows down the heart; slower heart means lower blood pressure.
- **Move your legs first.** Slow down your morning get ups; start with rotating your ankles and moving your feet up and down; this will push blood that has pooled up the legs.
- **Sit down.** Sit down when coughing; coughing slows down heart rate in the same way straining does, by activating the vagus nerve; put the shame aside, it is acceptable for males to sit down while peeing.

- **Lean forward.** If you start blacking out hold on to something and bend forward; this rushes the blood to the head giving you some extra time to sit down safely.

The precautions above will help you avoid accidents that can arise from sudden blood pressure, but they are not able to repair an underlying faulty blood pressure mechanism. For that you need to take a much wider angle.

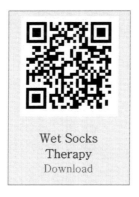

Wet Socks
Therapy
Download

http://goo.gl/3TT6g3

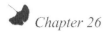 *Chapter 26*

An ortho that's late

Remember the ortho test you did in the earlier chapter? If your results were vague, but you felt worse, dizzy or faint *after* the test you want to read this chapter with utmost attention. This chapter will explain why swinging blood pressure may have such unpredictable patterns and what it means to health.

It's not healthy

Delayed orthostatic hypotension is a serious concern, not only because it indicates poor health, but also because it is commonly under-recognized. Delayed postural hypotension is not given sufficient attention despite suggestions that it may be linked to nervous system failure.

Current clinical setup rarely facilitates testing for a delayed blood pressure drop. The test requires sufficient space for performing it, special tilt table, and staff that continuously monitors the patient for thirty to forty-five minutes. Because of these difficulties the test is seldom performed and positives are seldom found. Yet despite infrequent diagnosis the problem is not rare at all. A study published in *Neurology* in 2006 found that a delayed blood pressure drop affected 54 % of tested individuals.[118]

Flawless automation is the key to health

The body is armed with multiple mechanisms guarding the stability of blood pressure. Hundreds and thousands of commands are orchestrated in the background without any input of our conscious mind. When performed flawlessly and synced appropriately these automatic processes keep blood pressure at the desired level regardless of exertion, movement, and emotional stress.

When these mechanisms fail, blood pressure fails to respond properly and stays at the mercy of automatic mechanisms coming on or off at unpredictable times. With faulty automation triggers no longer result in action, and stops get ignored. Imagine driving a car where neither breaks nor accelerators work when they need to, but activate themselves at random times.

This is exactly what happens with autonomic nervous failure. Body mechanisms turn themselves on at inappropriate times. Timely automation no longer exists. Blood pressure goes down during exercise, and up during sleep. Everything seems to be upside down, unpredictable, and random.

Autonomic nervous system failure is a big problem because all body functions, not only blood pressure, depend on it. Hormone secretion, carbohydrate metabolism, muscular reflexes, respiration, sexual arousal and digestion also rely heavily on the autonomic nervous system.

Signs of faulty automation

Autonomic failure does not happen overnight. It is a gradual process so elusive that few of us take notice. Erectile troubles, night-time urination, or fluctuating blood pressure are discussed separate problems and treatment is given separately for each. Very few clinicians look at the big picture and many patients falsely accept the symptoms as an inevitable part of aging.

Taking all these symptoms together can tell a different story, the story of a progressive degeneration and a need for better detection and prioritization of treatment. Who cares about a sticky keyboard when the entire computer motherboard is about to crash! For the same reason, why limit a treatment of a leaky bladder while the whole body automation risks failure?

Here is a short list of symptoms that may, but not always do, accompany malfunctioning automation. These can be insignificant signs of a significant problem.

- **Bladder** issues: having to pee at night, involuntary urination, lack of sensation of bladder fullness, stress incontinence (urine leaks on coughing or sneezing), urinary frequency without infection[119]
- **Sexual** issues: erectile troubles, impotence, lack of morning erection (!), difficulty with arousal and achieving orgasm, or untimely ejaculation
- **Bowel** problems: more frequent and less solid stools, chronic explosive diarrhea, uncontrollable farting (I do not mean teenagers), or diarrhea at night
- Changes in **sweating**: disappearance of sweating, especially on legs

Later signs may be more obvious and more concerning such as:

- Fainting after exercise
- Repeated light-headedness, weakness and easy fainting
- Increasingly fluctuating blood pressure
- Unsteady gait
- Slurring of speech
- Dimming of vision

Other signs that you may have noticed, but you did not think much of:

- Chronic one-sided nasal congestion[120]
- Daily headaches or migraines
- Cravings for sugar and/or salt
- Cardiac arrhythmia
- Different blood pressure readings on either arm

Let's say you have few of these symptoms. Should you be concerned?

Before making a mountain out of a molehill contact a licensed health practitioner first. You need a thorough checkup and proper diagnosis. Having the above symptoms does not automatically mean the problem is affecting multiple body systems and is stemming from autonomic system failure.

Second, take precautions to control your existing symptoms: adjust medication, hydrate better, and avoid sudden movements. You should also pay better attention to personal hygiene, open communication with the partner, and if necessary, remodel the house or get walking aid to improve mobility.

Third, take measures to prevent further decline of autonomic nervous system and better yet, put an extra effort to stimulate its regeneration. Don't expect that a short-term diet or a pill will do. For nervous system repair you will need to maintain continuous long-term effort and be under a supervision of a knowledgeable physician.

The best doctor to help you in your journey towards full body regeneration is a board-certified/licensed naturopathic doctor/physician or a physician trained in restorative medicine. Be aware, though, that different countries, states, and provinces have different laws and regulations. What's called an orange in one place may mean a plum or a goat in the other. In some places training and requirements for naturopathic doctors are at par or even higher than that of medical doctors. In some other places, though, a naturopathic doctor may mean a weekend-trained practitioner that never saw an anatomy book. Enquire so as not to be disappointed. But even though you may not have access to a well-trained holistic doctor there are a few things you can do on your own.

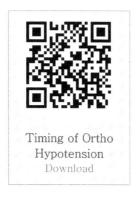

Timing of Ortho
Hypotension
Download

http://goo.gl/rhqjGx

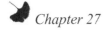 *Chapter 27*

Can I take a pill for that?

Before any restorative treatment is effective, though, one must ensure that the body has all the necessary nutrients for healing. The nervous system just like any other system in the body relies on nutrients that come from a diet.

But eating alone does not guarantee good nourishment. What and where one eats makes a difference. While processed food is known to be largely devoid of nutrients, homemade meals don't always provide full nutritional insurance. Even *un*processed produce may have inferior nutrient score due to depleted soil it is grown in.

There is also our birthdate. With age weakened digestion limits food choices and nutrient absorption. So even though we live in a land of plenty, malnutrition is common in our aging society. Add to it abundance of junk, reliance on processed food, wide-spread poor soil quality, diseases of digestive tract, food allergies, cultural and religious restrictions and we have a glaring problem.

Blood pressure irregularities and autonomic nervous system failure (dysautonomia) is largely aggravated by malnutrition. Multiple studies show that nutrient deficiencies may not only contribute, but also directly lead to nervous system degeneration.[121] Deficiencies of vitamin E, B, magnesium and many others nutrients are either directly or indirectly implicated in the process.

Below are the three most important nutrients needed for a flawless nervous system performance: vitamin B1, vitamin B12, and magnesium.

Vitamin B1

Deficiency of thiamin (vitamin B1) has been suggested as a possible frequent starting point of nervous system malfunction.[122] A widespread use of high carbohydrate meals and soft drinks seems to be, at least partially, responsible for triggering the problem. High sugar and high carb foods as well as drinks lower blood levels of this vitamin. People who crave and use sugars are at the highest risk of developing autonomic nervous system failure, which when advanced will lead to erratic blood pressure.[123]

Clinical symptoms of vitamin B1 deficiency, called beriberi, manifest as emotional instability, muscle loss, confusion, tingling in legs and hands, and sometimes swelling of ankles.[124] These symptoms are very common in the elderly. Although a complete depletion of vitamin B1 is rare nowadays, be aware that even a partial depletion can result in inadequate nervous system performance.

Levels of vitamin B1 are tested extremely rarely in clinical settings and you have close to zero chances of being informed about B1 stores. So instead of waiting for an unlikely B1 status diagnosis invest in a full spectrum B complex supplement. This will prevent or even deal with any already existing B vitamin deficiency.

Vitamin B12

Vitamin B12 is yet another well-known B vitamin the body needs for repair and regeneration of the nervous system. It is also necessary for maintaining cardiovascular function, including heart performance, arterial health, and blood flow. Yet vitamin B12 is one of the most common missing vitamins in people suffering from fatigue, anxiety, poor liver detoxification, and heart disease. Vitamin B12 levels, not unlike vitamin B1 levels, are seldom routinely tested and many people walk about with deficiency without realizing it.

There are two main groups most affected by deficiency of B12 vitamin: people with poor digestion and vegetarians. Vegetarians may show the deficiency already within a few months after starting the diet. Vegans are the biggest suspects as plant world does not have a good source of this vitamin.

But even those who are not opposed to eating meat are not guaranteed to be free of deficiencies and should test vitamin B12 levels routinely. Absorption of vitamin B12 is unusually elaborate and only people with the most robust digestive system can absorb sufficient amounts.

A B12 test is simple. It is a blood draw that can be ordered by any licensed doctor. No fasting required. But if you haven't been tested and prefer to skip the needle you should not leave matters alone and consider adding B12 to your supplement regimen as a nutritional insurance. Vitamin B12 is not toxic and if your body does not need it, it will excrete it without any side effects.

Consider taking this vitamin even though your doctor, who tested you, did not inform you of any B12 deficiency. Your doctor compares your numbers to established lab norms, which are set to diagnose *clinical deficiency*, not *optimal* body stores. And these are vastly different.

Lab numbers are not optimal

Optimal range is not set in stone, but every nutritionally oriented doctor can tell you that it is definitely different than the standard lab range. Clinical deficiency of vitamin B12 can be diagnosed when the levels fall below 148 pmol/L. But this level is set way below B12 needed for optimal performance. My clinical experience attests for that. Suggesting B12 to people who seemingly are not deficient has been shown to help many erase their symptoms such anxiety, toe tingling, fatigue, and forgetfulness.

Since your doctor may not be nutritionally trained and may not be able to distinguish between clinical deficiency and optimal stores do not assume that if you are told nothing your B12 deficiency, your vitamin levels are good. For the same reason do not assume that if you are not deficient as per lab norms, you automatically have optimal B12 stores. The difference between deficient and optimal is simple. Your body can survive, but it will not thrive. For optimal stores, aim to see vitamin B12 blood levels at 500 pmol/L or higher.

To be sure about your B12 level check the numbers yourself. Do not be afraid to ask your doctor to show you the blood work. You are entitled to it. It's your body. Twenty-five per cent of American adults have diagnosable clinical vitamin B12 deficiency.[125] And according to Statistics Canada over ninety-six per cent of Canadians have B12 above 148 pmol/L, but below optimal numbers.[126] It looks like many are surviving, but few are thriving.

Supplementing B12 is not as straightforward as swallowing a pill. Vitamin B12 tablets that are designed to be swallowed seldom work. It is also unlikely that you can absorb a sufficient amount of vitamin B12 from a multivitamin or a multi B tablet. Only injections, drops or sublingual tablets/strips that by-pass digestive system can adequately bump B12 reserves. Choose your supplements wisely, and definitely not because they are on sale.

Magnesium

Are you anxious, fatigued, and craving chocolate? Chances are you need magnesium. Magnesium controls nervous system excitability and it is crucial for energy and neurotransmitter production. Modern science strongly links magnesium deficiencies with nervous system disorders, including dysautonomia.[127] [128]

Magnesium deficiency is common in epilepsy, Alzheimer's, and Parkinson's disease. But confusion, disorientation, and depression can happen even with partial magnesium depletion. Lack of magnesium is a frequent contributor to muscle spasms and twitches, weakness, and bladder incontinence.[129]

Magnesium is found predominantly in dark green leafy vegetables, nuts and seeds, beans and lentils as well as whole grains. Despite wide availability of these foods it is not easy to satisfy daily its requirements.

Food content of magnesium has drastically declined since 1950. About three quarters of Americans eat magnesium-deficient diet.[130] It is not uncommon to see 25%-95% of magnesium reduction in many food sources.[131] For example, refining grains depletes them of 80-97% of this mineral. But even unprocessed food is not perfect. Collard greens have 84% less magnesium today than three decades ago due to soil changes as well as modern agricultural practices.

Our personal dietary choices may also add to already widespread magnesium deficiency. Pop, soda, sweets, and caffeine all deplete body stores of magnesium.[132] Frequent use of these magnesium robbers has a definite negative impact on body nutrient stores. Considering poor soil quality, nutrient-depleting food processing, and imperfect food choices magnesium deficiency likely applies to all of us.

Magnesium supplements come in variety of shapes and sizes. Your local health food store will be able to tailor magnesium supplement to your needs so plan to visit one in the near future.

Rethinking values

Many people inadvertently make dietary choices that contribute to ill-health and nutritional deficiencies. When buying food we think of convenience, price and taste, seldom of health or nutrient value. Faster and cheaper means better. We are well accustomed to fast take outs and ready-made deli counters. Life is busy, so why waste time on groceries, meal planning, and cooking.

But exactly this way of thinking is what gets us in a vicious cycle of busy life – poor food – ill health. Poor food may be cheap, but ill-health it results in will cost much more to repair. You may not give it a thought, but money saved on cheap "value" meals has short legs. Soon you may have to spend it on more expensive health correcting measures: supplements, doctors, and drugs. The financial drain poor nutrition causes continues indefinitely and only gets worse over time.

My Provencal soup

Many people think that eating out saves time and money. Even more people claim that they cannot afford organics. And the truth is that a $3.99 soup served at a fast food stand does not look expensive, but $4.99 for a small bunch of organic leeks surely will turn off many shoppers. With such a price difference are organic groceries even worth buying then?

Organics are the most nutrient dense foods one can buy. Organic produce is grown in nutrient-rich soil without use of man-made herbicides and pesticides. Organic produce is undoubtedly the purest and the most nourishing food available on the market, but does one have to be a millionaire to afford it?

I use mostly organics and many times I was questioning my choices. Am I jeopardizing my family finances because I buy expensive produce? Would we not be better off eating like everybody else? Should I trade the time spend in the kitchen for lining up in food places? Is the time and money worth the trouble at the end?

To put the end to my uncertainty I decided to make a comparison. I compared the cost of making an organic soup to a standard soup available in a fast food restaurant. I used a Provencal vegetable soup recipe I found in the stash of cookbooks in my library. The recipe called for about nine different vegetables, broth, wine, and spices. I bought them all in my local grocery store carefully noting the price for each item. The table below has all the details.

Provencal Vegetable Soup - cost

Grocery item	Cost per amount used
Butter, organic	$0.30
Carrots, organic	$0.30
Leeks, organic	$4.00
Celery, organic	$0.30
Thyme, organic	$0.30
White wine, organic	$5.00
Vegetable stock, organic	$2.70
Potatoes, non-organic	$2.70
Beans, canned non-organic	$1.40
Asparagus, fresh non-organic	$3.50
Squash, organic	$6.00
Spinach, organic	$2.50
Peas, frozen non-organic	$0.75
Lemon, organic	$0.50
Total cost (yielded 6 Liters)	**$30.55**
Cost per cup	**$1.27**

Notice that the dollar value is only for the amounts used and also that not all items I bought were organic. The grocery store did not have organic peas, beans or potatoes, so I had to get a non-organic variety. The grocery bill looked large, so was the total for the soup, but this is exactly where a more careful analysis is needed.

My creation yielded six liters of super thick hardy soup with over-abundant chunks of vegetables in it. The vegetables were not even floating. There was no room. The soup was that thick. Yet, this was not a culinary mishap. I like soups like that. They beat highly diluted cheap varieties of fast food soups. They eat like a meal and are equally satisfying. You don't need anything else.

My boys are big eaters, but twenty-four cups of food is not easy to gulp down in one day. The fridge kept the soup for the next three day as we enjoyed it without having to cook again or line up to get a cup of nutritionally-impoverished slipslops.

The taste was heavenly, which is exactly how I like it. With doubling the spice and wine I keep it simmering until vegetables give their juices up. Artificially-flavored mixture will never beat a real thyme and lemon flavor, at least according to my culinary preferences.

My time investment for twenty-four servings of soup was about one and a half hours, which includes time for grocery shopping, washing, peeling, as well as cooking. That is considerably less time than I would spend for driving up to a restaurant, lining up, and waiting to be served ready-to-eat meals for the next three days.

My financial investment for the soup was $30.55, which is $1.27 per serving. I am yet to find a place that serves an organic wine based soup, not colored water, for less than $1.50.

It does not matter how you look at it. Whether you consider nutrition, time, finances, convenience, or health effects the bottom line is the same: you can only benefit from switching from take outs to home cooked organic meals. Organic produce and home cooking may look expensive and inconvenient on the surface, but after analysis they are more time and cost effective than take-outs, while providing a much higher nutrition value for the body.

Before you reach for drugs or supplements to erase ailments ensure that you removed the likely cause of those: impoverished diet. What`s the point of popping pills to correct symptoms while the most obvious reason for those remains uncorrected?

Provencal Soup
Recipe
Download

http://goo.gl/nLQWCU

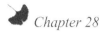 *Chapter 28*

Water does that too!

Is there a way to bring back strength to the nervous system, make the body resilient and tough without yet another diet, drug, or supplement? Yes, there is. It is a simple and old method used for centuries and it is the same method that boosted cardiovascular and immune system in the previous chapter – hydrotherapy.

Hydrotherapy does not fail even when it comes to dealing with the most difficult task: repairing faulty body automation. If done properly, water can provide just the right stimulus to organs and systems to get them back on track. Studies have shown that hydrotherapy can affect not only peripheral nervous system and circulation, but also production of hormones, digestion, respiration, bladder control, movement of lymphatics, and many aspects of the immune system. For example, a simple application of cold water can reduce edema and muscular pain and a warm compress applied to the back can double intestinal peristalsis and treat constipation.[133]

Rewriting the brain

Hydrotherapy effects are extremely powerful and it is said that repeated cold emersions could potentially restore normal function even in chronic fatigue syndrome.[134] Consider this being great news, because a pill, whether drug or supplement, for chronic fatigue syndrome is yet to be discovered.

Be prepared that your restorative cold hydrotherapy will not be pleasant. It takes guts and devotion to plunge into a frigid bath. However, once your emotions are dealt with you should expect cold hydrotherapy to be highly rewarding. Cold water effects are not limited to a temporary increase in energy. Cold water is also capable of reconditioning the brain.

Cold water stimulates hypothalamus-pituitary-adrenal axis, which is at the core of body automation.[135] Yes, those simple cold showers have a profound action on rebuilding the brain and the entire nervous system. They increase production of multiple hormones and neurotransmitters, without which execution of automation would not be possible.

You probably know two of those neurotransmitters already: beta-endorphin, famous for its pain reducing ability and cortisol known as a powerful inflammation quencher. Cold showers stimulate production of both, which makes water sort of like an aspirin minus its side effects. Cold showers relieve pain, reduce inflammation, and improve blood flow, but without giving stomach ulcers in return.

Norepinephrine for blood pressure

But what about erratic blood flow? Can water help with that? Sure it can! Repeated cold showers boost production of norepinephrine, a neurotransmitters responsible for adjustment in blood pressure.[136] Norepinephrine's job is to keep blood pressure steady and prevent blood pressure from dropping[137] exactly what you want to prevent excessively fluctuating blood pressure.

Norepinephrine is produced "on demand." Its job is to send a "get ready" message to the blood vessels when the body needs to adjust blood pressure upwards. The command is received by the small muscles surrounding the arteries. They tighten up and as a result blood vessels narrow. This raises blood pressure. The muscles will keep firm till the command "relax" arrives. Only then blood vessels open and blood pressure naturally drops.

When norepinephrine is lacking, arterial muscles do not get a toning stimulus. They do not tighten up and do not keep blood vessels compressed. When one stands up suddenly blood pressure drops instead of going up. Dropping blood pressure leads to insufficient blood flow to the brain and that leads to light-headedness and appearance of stars (I don't mean celebrities).

Boosting your own norepinephrine production

In medicine, supplementation of norepinephrine is not common, although norepinephrine can be used to treat hypotension. Norepinephrine is not a pill. It is an injection and it is given usually in emergency situations under doctor's supervision. It is not a treatment given out frequently and it is reserved only for the most severe cases of low blood pressure.[138]

A well-functioning body should have its own sufficient on-demand supply of norepinephrine. But not all bodies are capable of delivering squirts of norepinephrine on time and in the right quantity. Aging and weak adrenals can contribute to that.

In an ideal world norepinephrine is produced quickly and sufficiently to satisfy the changing body demands. The bulk of this production happens in the adrenals, glands located above the kidneys. These, however, carry a burden of our stressful modern lifestyle. Hectic lifestyles can cause adrenal fatigue and weakened adrenals may lag in satisfying norepinephrine demands of the body.

Adrenal restoration is not a one-day treatment. It may take weeks or months to see perfectly satisfactory results. But don't give up! You still can help your failing blood pressure today even though your adrenals may be chronically "busted" from living a hectic life. The only thing you need to do is to muster the courage and grit to get your cold showers daily. That will start norepinephrine going.

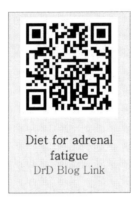

Diet for adrenal
fatigue
DrD Blog Link

http://goo.gl/77ogHG

Chapter 29

Stronger lives longer

Let's go back to ortho results. You may recall that they were divided into five categories. The first category referred to people who ended up with an increase of blood pressure. You already know what a decrease means, but you may be wondering what it means if blood pressure actually goes up. Is this a good thing or did one suddenly develop hypertension.

Many broadly-trained clinicians use orthostatic tests as a measure of nervous system stability and adrenal health. For those whose aim is to strengthen neuro-hormonal feedback an increase in blood pressure after standing can actually mean a good thing.

Blood pressure as a health marker

If you read the earlier chapter attentively it could become obvious to you that standing up should never result in a blood pressure drop. Healthy individuals are expected to produce a robust amount of norepinephrine to keep blood pressure steady, even when challenged. Healthy circulation should not lead to dizziness even with vigorous exercise because blood pressure is capable of adjusting with every move, going up and down as needed. This quick and error-free blood pressure regulation is something to hold on to because it reflects good health.

Just as a drop in blood pressure matches poorer health, a sizable increase in blood pressure shortly after standing up is a welcomed sign. When the nervous system is fully functional and the circulatory system is highly responsive, the body is able not only to compensate for the gravity shift, but also can anticipate and attempt to prevent any additional circulatory stress.

The internal blood pressure balancing is not an easy task. To be perfectly executed the body has to get through many steps. First it has to send a rapid feedback about changes to blood flow, then propagate a corrective command along the nerves, then activate tiny muscles located on blood vessels, and then check again if the desired effect is achieved. If blood pressure is not where it should be the cycle repeats. The pathways are complicated and there is quite a room for error. This multi-step task of blood pressure adjustment is carried out perfectly only in truly healthy individuals.

Ortho guide to adrenals

A perfectly working nervous system and adrenals are able to recover from postural changes and restore blood pressure completely within a few seconds.[139] An increase of blood pressure upon standing is a well-anticipated response for healthy adrenals.[140] But that does not mean the higher the better. Not every generous increase is good. Blood pressure that goes over 20 points is not considered healthy any more.[141] The most desirable orthostatic outcome is an increase of systolic number by 6-10 mmHg. Such a moderate spike has been suggested as an indicator of well-functioning adrenals, which, as you will learn shortly, is a prerequisite for good health.

Below is a quick guide explaining how ortho test is used for estimating adrenal performance.[142]

Systolic (top number) behavior on standing	*Approximate adrenal function estimation*
Increases more than 10 mmHg	*Strong, but overactive adrenals*
Increases 6-10 mmHg	*Good adrenal function*
Does not change	*Fair adrenal function*
Drops 1-10 mmHg	*Poor adrenal function*
Drops more than 10 mmHg	*Adrenal exhaustion*

Adrenals key to good health

Adrenals are not just any organ. They regulate body automation and decide on overall quality of life for that matter. Adrenals are so essential that even Traditional Chinese Medicine (TCM) established thousands of years ago had something to say about their importance. TCM does not recognize adrenals as a separate organ, but since adrenals rest on kidneys they are simply considered part of a "kidney complex."

In TCM, "kidneys" carry the essence of life and it is said that once the essence is gone, so is life. Hair graying, back pain, ear noises, involuntary ejaculation, leg swelling, fatigue, infertility, poor memory, dizziness, poor eyesight, tooth and bone loss are signs that kidney essence is weak. In TCM, kidneys govern birth, growth, reproduction and development and thus are the most important body organs, organs that govern vitality and lifespan.

Despite the fact that modern medicine does not consider TCM as a compelling source of medical information it cannot disagree that adrenals are the keys to good health. You may know from previous chapters that adrenals produce norepinephrine that regulates blood pressure, but science has found out that adrenals' job is not limited to doing just that one task. Their job is way bigger than regulating blood pressure. Adrenals regulate functions of the entire body. Adrenals are involved in blood sugar regulation, lipid metabolism, growth, inflammation, electrolyte balance, sexual response, hormone production, fight and flight and countless other functions, so their role is exceptionally vital.

Time to look up to ancient wisdom

TCM is yet to find acceptance among western sceptics. Decades of abolished rejections, doubts, objections, discussions, and counterarguments were needed to elevate acupuncture from useless sham to a medical treatment status. Understandably, due to their narrowly defined paradigm, it was simply too difficult for medical researchers to comprehend how a seemingly "random" needling of skin may produce any effect on organs, hormones, or neurotransmitters. It sounded weird that needling a hand would have an effect on the bowels, and needling a foot could change liver function.

Despite current widespread acceptance of acupuncture our western medical system is still cautious about other "unfounded" eastern concepts that "lack evidence." Western medicine never looked into and has no plans to use TCM philosophy as a springboard to accelerate and deepen the understanding of human physiology. After all, TCM does not base its diagnosis and treatment on lab values, but on body energetics, a concept foreign and still considered as silly by many western doctors.

But guess what! The ancient wisdom may not have been sucked out of thin air as some people think. As science is making progress in understanding body physiology we are getting convinced that eastern philosophy presents a valuable insight. The concept that "kidneys" hold the key to long life known to Chinese doctors for thousands of years has specifically been confirmed by modern science just now. A far-fetched idea that "kidneys" hold the essence of life is no longer an "absurd" or "bunk," but a scientifically confirmed correlation between adrenal function, health, and longevity.

Several recent studies found that DHEA, a hormone produced by adrenals may serve as a marker for longevity.[143,144] DHEA, a precursor of multiple hormones, declines with age, but its decline varies among individuals and depends on adrenal output.

Think of DHEA as a grandfather of other hormones. Estrogen, testosterone, cortisol, pregnenolone, and growth hormone all come from DHEA. They orchestrate our behavior and disease patterns. Low DHEA leads to inflammation, insulin resistance, poor immunity, infertility, frailty, poor memory, and poor circulation. Low DHEA is associated with heart disease, atherosclerosis, osteoporosis, and sexual problems among many others.[145]

Declining DHEA leads to declining of health, marks the end of robustness and starts the onset of frailness. Weakening of adrenals is echoed by general deterioration, and that includes meager orthostatic blood pressure behavior.

Maybe it is time all doctors take orthostatic test to heart and use it as a marker for general health, not just a time-consuming nuisance experiment. Let's not wait another thousand years before new official health guidelines are posted. They may come a tad too late.

DHEA + Adrenal
Test
Link to Store

http://goo.gl/ZE7fKW

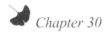 *Chapter 30*

What if you have adrenal fatigue?

Since adrenal fatigue is not recognized by the orthodox medical system don't expect to get this diagnosis from your traditionally trained medical doctor. Do not expect your doctor either to use the ortho test to measure your adrenals. For an endocrinologist to intervene you will need to have a total adrenal exhaustion, called Addison`s disease, a condition that has to be confirmed by blood work.

Adrenal fatigue is extremely common in our fast-paced, highly stressed society. Daily pressures, business worries, challenging relationships, difficult working conditions all contribute to adrenal stress. Here is a short list of most common modern contributors to adrenal fatigue:

- Chronic inflammation, chronic pain
- Sleep deprivation, shift work, poor sleeping habits
- Ongoing cumulative environmental toxicity
- Chronic illness, chronic allergies, chronic infections
- Overwork, mental and physical strain
- Trauma, injury, surgery, over-exercise
- Hypoglycemia, starvation, not eating on time
- Poor diet, mal-digestion, mal-absorption, nutritional deficiencies
- Frustration, anger, depression, fear, guilt

Adrenal fatigue is difficult to diagnose, because it does not result in drastically low blood hormone values, which is the case with Addison's disease, but it manifest itself in variety of fashions and mimic other diseases and conditions. Here are common findings suggestive of adrenal fatigue:

- Chronic fatigue, poor memory, "senior moments," confusion, low concentration
- Loss of sex drive
- Cravings for salt and sweets, excessive hunger, alcohol intolerance
- Recurrent infections
- Chronic inflammation or pain
- Inability to handle stress
- Low blood pressure, fluctuating blood pressure, dizziness on standing
- Weakness, low body temperature
- Anxiety, nervousness, apprehension, irritability, insomnia
- Dry, thin skin
- Osteoporosis

In the next chapter you will learn how to help your adrenals. Although bringing adrenals back to their full power requires medical expertise you can do a lot of good just by following the simple breathing technique described in the next pages.

This technique will benefit both the overactive as well as the underactive adrenals, so regardless where you stand on the ortho test you can't go wrong.

http://goo.gl/Mvg2i1

Foods for
Adrenals
Download

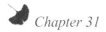 *Chapter 31*

The art of breathing

Have you ever noticed that running and slow breathing do not go well together? Have you ever tried to fall asleep while panting? This does not go well either.

Breathing rate is intimately tied in to level of excitement. These two always go together. Breath paces nervous system and nervous system dictates the breath rate. Excitement speeds up breathing, and stillness slows it down. The opposite is true as well. Slow breathing calms down the nerves and fast breathing excites. Now it is clear that your breath must be slow when you sleep and fast when you jog.

Because of that interdependence your breath is capable of telling your nervous system when to get excited and when to relax. You can use that knowledge to your advantage, and specifically to work with adrenals.

Failing adrenals are adrenals that have been long under chronic stress. You need to reduce stress before attempting to rebuild them. I know, you cannot make bills disappear, turn kids into angels, and have your business triple customers overnight, but you can cheat the stress with breath. It is true—you can reduce the anxiety and frustration within minutes by slowing down the respiration.

Breathe like a pro: belly, nose, slow!

First, you need to breathe from your belly, not the chest. You need to master abdominal breathing well for it to be effective. Use a mirror to see how you breathe. Most people I know are chest breathers. Chances are you are too.

Why is abdominal breathing important? Because only abdominal breathing can calm the nerves down. Chest breathing accomplishes the opposite. It causes more stress. Studies showed that chest breathing stimulates fight-and-flight response by activating branches of sympathetic nervous system.[146] Chest breathers not only get less oxygen, but also get more stressed. Remember to use your belly. Always.

Second, ensure to breathe through your nose, not through the mouth. The nose contains a special apparatus that helps activate relaxation response. This magic happens in paranasal sinuses. As air passes through the sinuses they produce nitric oxide.[147] Nitric oxide causes vasodilation, blood vessel relaxation.[148] Due to this effect nitric oxide is considered a major cardiovascular player protecting against heart failure, high blood pressure, strokes, and ischemia (oxygen insufficiency).[149]

Third, slow down your breath to an unhurried six per minute. Six breaths per minute is equivalent to taking a new breath every ten seconds. Five seconds for inhalation and another five for exhalation. Studies showed that this natural rhythm is capable of not only producing a feeling relaxation, but also general improvement in health.

To appreciate the importance of rhythmical breathing it is sufficient to say that is it *"synchronises inherent cardiovascular rhythms and modify baroreflex sensitivity."*[150] In lay language it means slow rhythmical breathing helps cardiac patients live longer. Interestingly, reciting Ave Maria prayer and yoga mantra results in rhythmical six breaths per minute. Maybe that's why people who go to church at least once a week extend the lifespan by seven years.[151]

There is much more to say about six breaths per minute. The technique seems to strongly enhance heart rate variability.[152] Heart rate variability (HRV) is a time interval between heart beats. Ample HRV parallels good health and low HRV is associated with poor prognosis.

Heart rate variability decreases when the person is under emotional strain and in the state of anxiety.[153] Low HRV predicts heart attacks and is associated with numerous ailments including diabetic neuropathy. HRV is also a very strong marker for autonomic nervous system strength,[154] which ties in to adrenals and blood pressure behavior.

Since you have to breathe you may as well learn to do it like a pro. Use your belly and your nose, not the chest or your mouth. Slow down to six per minute. Practice while stuck in traffic, before a dental appointment, during stressful meetings, or before giving a speech. Breathe right to restore the adrenals, regulate blood pressure, and before meals to enhance digestion.

Breathing right will not only help you escape stress, but also regulate another possible blood pressure irregularity: POTS.

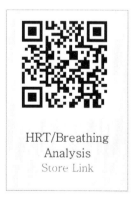

HRT/Breathing
Analysis
Store Link

http://goo.gl/QmyBZz

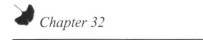 *Chapter 32*

POTS, but not for cooking

POTS is an acronym for Postural Orthostatic Tachycardia Syndrome, a fancy medical name given to a speedy heart rate. POTS is a recent addition to a medical dictionary which describes an exceptionally racy heart during the standing up test you I described before.

Postural Orthostatic Tachycardia Syndrome applies only to adults as kids have a much faster heart rate to begin with. Suspect that you have POTS if your heart rate accelerated over thirty beats per minute while doing the ortho test.[155] A modest acceleration of a heart rate on standing is normal and desirable, but too much of a good thing is never right.

Palpitations, fatigue, headaches?

Postural Orthostatic Tachycardia Syndrome can lead to palpitations, light-headedness, shortness of breath, and weakness. Some people with POTS may experience blurry vision and even lose consciousness. It is frequent in migraineurs and POTS may even aggravate the headaches. Forty-eight per cent of people with POTS have fatigue and thirty-two per cent suffer from sleep problems.[156]

One interesting symptom of POTS is redness of feet and purplish/blotchy skin. This is due to blood pooling in the legs. For a sedentary person this skin discoloration usually does not cause other symptoms except aesthetic concerns. But for those who spend time in the gym blood pooling in legs may lead to heart fluttering or unsteadiness during exercise.

Postural Orthostatic Tachycardia Syndrome is five to ten times more common than orthostatic hypotension.[157] But POTS is not just yet another scary cardiovascular disease to worry about. It is a condition frequently caused by lifestyle factors such as dehydration and physical deconditioning. Since by now you are an expert in hydration this cause of POTS you can easily manage. Getting rid of the other cause of POTS, deconditioning, requires some explanation.

Deconditioning

The definition of deconditioning goes like this: *"Deconditioning is adaptation of an organism to less demanding environment, or, alternatively, the decrease of physiological adaptation to normal conditions."* In other words, a deconditioned body cannot take challenges because it is less adaptable to changes. In people with POTS deconditioning manifests as heart racing upon standing. Over-exaggerated beating of the heart is nothing else but an excessive compensation for a relatively small physical stress. Such reaction is rare in well-conditioned and fit individuals.

Deconditioning is a common occurrence in modern societies. North Americans do not fit into a picture of athleticism. With three quarters being overweight or obese we cannot say that North Americans are a population of fitness models. Conveniences, cars, elevators, escalators, scooters, and deliveries do not help with this predicament. The basics of living such as transportation, meal preparation, and communication require no physical effort.

We no longer need to carry heavy logs, chop wood, and hunt to get a meal. It's enough to click or dial and food magically appears at the door. Saddling a horse or climbing a wagon is no longer needed either. One can see a friend or attend a meeting also just by entering a sequence into a keyboard.

Since there is no longer any need for physical rigor, except finger dexterity, deconditioning is a natural, although not desirable, end-result. It is unfortunate, but modern life can leave us physically weakened in a short time.

Deconditioning is a well-documented phenomenon accompanying periods of physical dormancy. It can be especially pronounced after a period of bed rest or in other words periods of "doing nothing".[158] Bed rest, which is not always voluntary and can be a result of illness or accident, causes substantial changes in body reflexes. During bed rest the heart muscle adapts to lack of effort, becomes less ambitious and pumps smaller volume.[159]

Bed rest is not different from the chair rest many of us suffer from. The biggest difference between the two is that the first one is usually *in*voluntary and is *caused by* a health breakdown, whereas the other one is voluntary and *causes* health breakdown.

A sedentary lifestyle is a well-known primal culprit behind modern deconditioning phenomenon. But is it affecting you as well? Here is a quick test: if waking upstairs leaves you huffing and puffing and jogging is out of the question you are quite advanced in the deconditioning process.

Now imagine this scenario. A person with low or fluctuating blood pressure and little physical conditioning falls ill: flu, fever, sweats and pain. What happens? Blood pressure goes down, palpitations up, and fluctuations become more notable.

How much longer would it be for such person to recover from "the virus" in comparison to a well-conditioned person? Of course much longer. This is why people with low blood pressure must engage in strenuous physical fitness on a regular basis or they risk an encounter with a mysterious never-to-go-away "chronic fatigue virus" AKA prolonged deconditioning experience.

Need to go physical

You may not want to hear it, but physical exertion and rigor is a must for maintaining a healthy heart. There is no way around it, so you may as well embrace it. Dust off that bicycle, check out that aqua class, and maybe go rowing. All these three physical activities can help you get back to a conditioning state without causing an additional havoc to blood pressure.

Avoid activities with excessive jumping, sudden position shifts, and aerobic classes until your heart feels stronger. Excessive cardiovascular stress caused by quick full-body movements is not for low and fluctuating blood pressure individuals. Not all intense types of exercise are good for the heart and some may make matters worse. Returning to a conditioning state is very individual. For best results seek the assistance of a kinesiologist or a fitness trainer knowledgeable in various circulatory conditions.

Don't avoid exercise because it does not feel right or makes you feel weak. It is not the exercise that is bad; it is your body that needs to get better. Challenge yourself. Only challenging activities will bring your body back to strength. Lack of physical challenge is the fastest road to physical deconditioning.

But why should you bother with regular exercise if fitness modelling isn't in your cards? Why should you waste time on push-ups and lifts if strength is not what you care for? After, all car, phone, and Internet do not require any.

Here is the reason: deconditioning has been shown to promote faulty body automation and that, you know, underlies the function of nervous, immune, digestive, respiratory, endocrine, and circulatory system.[160] Lack of sufficient nervous system challenges invariably leads to poorer reflexes and poorer overall body performance. Nobody expects a pianist to perform perfectly after a year of vacation, so why would anybody expect a heart to be in peak condition without challenging it to a physical rigor?

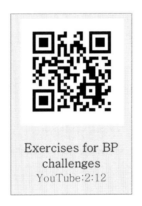

Exercises for BP
challenges
YouTube:2:12

https://youtu.be/bB_Zmysh3ZI

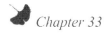 *Chapter 33*

Keep it at 40 even when older

A blood pressure monitor can indeed provide a wealth of knowledge about the body. Fluctuations during exertion, night dipping, morning cortisol awake, and orthostatic test may sound like a lot, but there is still more to discover. Although, I am not going to make you a cardiologist and get into complicated details of heart function there is still one circulatory parameter you should know about: pulse pressure.

Pulse pressure is calculated from your regular blood pressure readings. There is no need for additional testing equipment or even standing up. Pulse pressure is easily calculated from blood pressure taken at rest.

Introduction to pulse pressure

First let's see how healthy your pulse pressure is. Look back at your earlier blood pressure measurements. Locate one of your resting readings. Have the top and the bottom number in front of you for calculation. Now deduct the bottom number from the top one. The resulting number is your pulse pressure.

A healthy heart will keep pulse pressure at 40; a heart in trouble will keep it consistently either too high or too low. Pulse pressure over 40 is a warning sign of a malfunctioning circulation and pulse pressure over 60 may be used as a risk for cardiovascular disease.[161]

When pulse pressure is high

Changes to pulse pressure are common and they may be your first clues as to an improperly functioning cardiovascular system. Pulse pressure can point to already existing atherosclerosis, because the most common reason for an increased pulse pressure is stiffening of the arteries.

Healthy arteries are elastic and they accommodate changes in blood flow, but atherosclerotic arteries, arteries that have cholesterol and calcium deposits on their walls cannot do that. They are rigid. They cannot expand. They are narrow and stiff and cannot buffer circulatory peaks. Because of that loss of elasticity, clogged arteries produce a wide pulse pressure.

Pulse pressure that is consistently above 40 should definitely draw your attention. Studies showed that wide pulse pressure points to heart in need. A large study performed in 2000 on 8,000 patients revealed that for every ten point pulse pressure increase there is a 20 % increase in cardiovascular complications, which unfortunately includes cardiovascular deaths.[162] This correlation does not exclude people whose pulse pressure widens from use of medication.

If pulse pressure goes up due to arterial deposits major lifestyle habits changes are necessary. Make room for diet consisting of unprocessed organic foods, regular exercise, stress reduction, sunshine, and fresh air. Although this may be a large undertaking those who hesitate to plunge into changes can still make a difference by taking just one pill.

Folic acid, a popular vitamin, turns out to be a safe and effective method for curbing large pulse pressure. A study published in *American Journal of Clinical Nutrition* revealed that even a short-term supplementation of folic acid can produce a visible difference. In that study consumption of 5mg for three weeks resulted in a five point reduction of pulse pressure in a high percentage of individuals.[163] Folic acid does it by reducing arterial deposits and returning arteries to a more elastic state.

Five pressure points may not sound like much, but even this small change is worth aiming for when you consider that wide pulse pressure besides being implicated in heart disease is also linked to strokes[164] and dementia.[165]

Below 30?

Wide pulse pressure is no longer a mystery. It indicates heart disease and arterial hardening, but do you know where a *narrow* pulse pressure come from?

Let's start with pharmaceuticals. Certain prescription drugs, such as ACE inhibitors, a type of blood pressure medication, can artificially narrow pulse pressure.[166] Do not jump in excitement though. ACE inhibitors aren't the same as folic acid pills. They do not lower pulse pressure by cleaning the arteries from cholesterol deposits. ACE inhibitors do not reduce pulse pressure by making arteries more flexible, elastic and youthful, but by cutting off communication between nervous system and blood vessels.

ACE inhibitors are not the only one making changes to pulse pressure. Diuretics and other anti-hypertensive pills can do that as well. In fact, any medication, not only blood pressure drugs, may alter pulse pressure numbers. If you are on some sort of meds your pulse pressure may not reflect your actual cardiovascular situation.

But lower pulse pressure may not only come from medication. It can come from an internal problem. Smaller pulse pressure is a result of inadequate heart pumping, which can either reflect feeble nervous system signal, malfunctioning heart muscle or simply insufficient blood volume.

You already know the basics of strengthening the nervous system and by now you are an expert on hydration. And although you won't be able to repair everything that ails you without seeing a doctor you can still do a lot for your heart with home methods.

One of the causes of low blood volume you can address yourself is chronic blood loss. Low blood and pulse pressure can be caused by insufficient amount of circulating blood. To bump up the volume you need to detect and remedy hidden sources of blood loss, which is a topic of the next chapter.

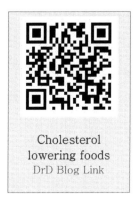

Cholesterol
lowering foods
DrD Blog Link

http://goo.gl/QKCDWs

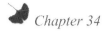 *Chapter 34*

What if there is not enough blood?

Have you ever gotten into a scuffle, fallen from a tree or tripped over a rock? Have you scraped yourself or end up with an open wound?

Regardless of the size of the trauma, you can detect blood loss with ease. Although minor blood loss is not of consequence, a more serious wound can cause symptoms. Hemorrhage cause weakness and dizziness within minutes.

For women only

Despite our "milder" nature and all safety precautions we take, women seem to be more prone than men to "bleeding accidents." We cannot change it. Nature designed it this way.

Regular monthly periods and the associated blood loss is nothing minor. Did you know that an average woman loses about three tablespoon of blood during that time and women with heavy menses can lose more than six tablespoons of the vital fluid? [167] Although that amount looks insignificant when compared to the blood volume in the entire body, it still can make a difference to blood pressure.

Anemia is one of the leading causes for hypotension. About 10% of North Americans are anemic, that's one out of ten.[168] However, women are ten times more prone to anemia than men. As you may have guessed the reason is lack of menses in males. Only one out of fifty males suffers from iron deficiency anemia, but as many as one out of five women can be drained by it.[169]

Iron pills are not for everyone

Paleness of skin, tongue, or gums can be a giveaway sign of anemia, but unless you are sure about its cause, do not medicate yourself with iron. Before heading to a health food store or a pharmacy ensure that your body actually needs this mineral. There are many different causes of anemia and iron deficiency is only one of them. You need to confirm that iron supplements can correct it, otherwise you will only end up frustrated.

Ask your doctor for blood test called "ferritin." It is a test that measures iron stores in the body. Medicating with iron when iron storage is normal can result in serious health problems. Iron can worsen inflammation and weaken the immune system.[170] It can even damage the liver. For that reason take iron supplements only when ferritin is low.

Think before going in circles

Starting on iron pills with low ferritin is no brainer, but what should you do if you continue staying low despite taking iron supplements? Do you need to continue taking iron if low ferritin and anemia do not want to go away?

Einstein once said "continuing doing the same thing over and over again and expecting a different result… that's insanity." So, let's apply Einstein's wisdom here: if a month or three on iron did not boost ferritin levels and anemia keeps on persisting you must change the strategy or you'll be going in circles. Reassess the cause or move to another treatment.

Unfortunately, long-term iron supplementation, despite poor results, is a common practice among health practitioners. I am puzzled as to why such routine treatment is so popular. It is not only ineffective, but also carries side effects that range from digestive upset to immune impairment. Continuous loading with iron in hope that one day iron stores somehow change their mind and magically go up is a plain absurd.

Look a bit further

Iron requires a well-acidified stomach and the presence of multiple other nutrients to be absorbed and incorporated in hemoglobin. If you continue to battle long-term anemia despite taking iron supplements you need to rethink the approach. Maybe the stomach does not have enough stomach acid or maybe iron assisting nutrients are missing.

To swiftly resolve chronic anemia, aim to work with a physician advanced in nutrition and knowledgeable in hematology. It is not impossible to turn chronic anemia into a three-month project under the eye of an expert doctor. But if finding such is difficult or if you prefer to work on your own I suggest that you start by checking a broader spectrum of nutrients, because building red blood cells is not limited to iron alone.

Red blood cells need a full range of vitamins and minerals including vitamin A, B12, folic acid, copper, and phosphorus. But a blood test is inadequate for nutritional assessment. Your doctor cannot tell if you need more calcium by scanning your blood test results. Minerals, except for iron, are difficult to test in blood. For that, hair analysis is a much better option. Hair analysis can be done through a licensed naturopathic doctor.

Hair analysis, in my opinion, is one of the better tool for assessing mineral reserves and their proportions. But to get accurate results your hair analysis has to be done by a specialized lab. Only accredited labs ensure consistent quality, minimize errors, and avoid misinterpretations. Hair analysis can inform you about the most important to human health minerals including iron, selenium, sulfur, manganese, magnesium, and chromium. Consider having hair analysis done regardless whether you have anemia or not. You never know. You may encounter a few unforeseen nutritional surprises.

Minor leaks, major problem

If you are concerned about low iron stores and already ruled out bleeding as a cause, here are a few additional factors that may block ferritin from climbing:

- Your **diet is iron deficient**. That is especially true in vegetarians and vegans; unless you become an omnivore you may need to add iron supplementation to your menu.
- Your **stomach is too alkaline**. Heartburn is a most common indicator of low stomach acidity; lemon juice is a good remedy to restore it.
- You are on **medication** that prevent or reduce iron absorption. Acid blockers are common ones; these are typically given for heartburn. Do not be afraid to question necessity or appropriateness of your medications; if you find that they are only managing symptoms you may want to switch to therapy that actually builds your health.
- Your **diet blocks iron absorption**. Heavy tea and milk use can do that; reduce tea and dairy products or use them away from main meals.
- You have **chronic bleeding**; find the blood leaks.

Where are those leaks?

Finding the source of chronic blood loss is not a difficult task, but first you must be aware of its existence. Chronic bleeding may be hidden and may neither hurt nor be obvious. Yet despite lack of discomfort don`t ignore its possibility, because even a loss of few drops a day can turn you into a white ghost over time.

Here are common situations that contribute to chronic blood loss. Ask a health professional to help you confirm those.

- Bleeding hemorrhoids (an external and internal exam may be needed)
- Fissures and fistulas within digestive system (they may not hurt, only a doctor can tell)
- Nicked colon polyps (you may need colonoscopy)
- Recurrent bladder infections (pee does not have to look pink)
- Micro-bleeding in urine for other reasons e.g. bladder cancer (urine dipstick test can help)
- Spotting between menses (check your panties regularly)
- Bleeding gums (check spit for reddish color)
- Stomach ulcers (they may not hurt if you are on painkillers)
- Daily use of aspirin and other anti-inflammatory drugs that irritate stomach mucosa (a risk factor for everyone)
- Blood thinning medication and supplements that prevent quick clotting (check skin for easy bruising)
- Micro-bleeding in faeces for other reasons such as colon cancer (ask your doctor for occult blood test in stool)

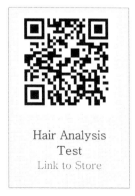

Hair Analysis
Test
Link to Store

http://goo.gl/hZPbyO

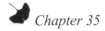 *Chapter 35*

Sugar boost, but no cakes!

Have you ever felt hungry to a point of a headache or body shaking? The chances are it was a hypoglycemia bout. Hypoglycemia is a fancier name for low blood sugar. Hypoglycemia is a commonly overlooked cause for hypotension.

Hypoglycemia, despite a prevalent belief, is not reserved to diabetics. It is a very common but under-recognized phenomenon in North America. The word "hypoglycemia" actually can cause confusion among practitioners, because it means a different thing to a traditionally trained medical doctor and emergency personnel then to a practitioner trained in functional medicine.

Hypoglycemia is not the same a hypoglycemia?!

In an emergency ward diagnosis of hypoglycemia is a serious matter. There is no time for errors, arguments, or uncertainty. Hypoglycemia, if not treated immediately, can lead to permanent brain damage, or even death. Therefore for medical personnel hypoglycemia has a precise lab cut off point. This is to prevent any confusion and facilitate prompt resuscitation.

Doctors are trained to recognize hypoglycemia when blood glucose falls below 3 mmol/L (54 mg/dl). This is a severe blood sugar drop, which typically is accompanied by extreme symptoms such as sweating, fainting, and stupor. Such type of hypoglycemia is mostly affecting diabetics using sugar lowering medication, especially insulin. Hypoglycemia of this kind is always a medical emergency.

However some health professionals use the word "hypoglycemia" differently. According to these doctors "hypoglycemia" is not limited to emergency situations, but also includes a relatively mild drop of blood sugar. This type of hypoglycemia does not result in a coma, neither it has an emergency lab range attached to it. It simply describes a state of insufficient blood glucose for optimal body function. This milder version of hypoglycemia has a completely different clinical presentation and requires a completely different treatment.

Today informing patients of their blood sugar irregularities presents a challenge as two different school of thoughts intercept. It is absolutely possible to be given up with two different diagnoses by two different doctors due to confused meaning of a word. However, as long as you know you that there are two different schools of thought, two different meanings behind the same word you will not be perplexed or frustrated.

Symptoms of low sugar

Although hypoglycemia is a known cause for low blood pressure, one does not have to reach an emergency state for blood pressure to get a nose dive. Sensitive individuals can register a change in blood pressure even with a small blood sugar drop. Those individuals will not have obvious emergency-type symptoms, but instead will notice minor changes in feeling of well-being.

Because diagnosable hypoglycemia must be confirmed by low blood sugar numbers the symptoms of milder non-emergency hypoglycemia do not usually fit the diagnostic lab profile. This is a source of confusion for many conventionally trained doctors that may be tempted to either completely disregard the symptoms or diagnose them as something else.

The reality is that an exceptionally large number of people walk about with minor blood sugar irregularities and symptoms of low blood sugar without realizing it. They are far from suspecting any blood sugar imperfections thinking that if they don't have diabetes there is nothing else in blood sugar department to pay attention to.

Mild hypoglycemia abounds with symptoms. Some are listed below. Look at them carefully, especially if you are overweight or underweight. A change in weight may be the first signal of blood sugar trouble.

- Sugar cravings
- Fatigue, low energy, see-sawing energy during the day
- Light-headedness, feeling of being spaced out
- Insomnia, difficulty falling asleep or staying asleep
- Temper tantrums, anger, easy frustration
- Anxiety, nervousness, irritability
- Hyperactivity, restlessness, impatience
- Cold hands and feet, body coldness
- Recurrent headaches
- Short attention span
- Forgetfulness, brain fog
- Low physical and mental performance

Oops! I have the symptoms!

Don't try to check your blood sugar whereabouts when you have these symptoms. Most likely the numbers will be in the "normal" range. As I said previously, don't be confused by it. If the symptoms are corrected by eating sugar chances are your body was low on fuel.

If you found out that your blood sugar fluctuates, you would need to correct it before your blood pressure can stabilize. It is low blood sugar that leads to low blood pressure, not the other way around. Your attention in that matter can really pay off.

Some people think that in order to correct low blood sugar one has to eat more sugar. This may be true in acute situation such as medication induced hypoglycemia, but this is not a treatment of choice for chronically low glucose. In fact, eating sugar can further disrupt glucose metabolism. Chronic tendency to low blood sugar is *not* corrected by eating cakes in a hurry, but by planning well-balanced meals ahead of time.

A permanent correction of symptoms related to hypoglycemia requires a smart nutritional strategy. The good news is that the steps to correct it are simple:

- Eat only small meals; snack rather than eat; this will prevent insulin surges that happen after large meals
- Eat frequently, every two to four hours; this will prevent in-between meal sugar dips
- Choose protein, fat and/or fiber rich meals; these keep sugar steady
- Avoid sweet drinks, including any fruit juices; they are very disruptive to blood sugar
- Avoid sugar substitutions; use normal sugar, but limit portions
- Let go of cakes, cookies, and other sugary junk; they are low blood sugar magicians; they can make hypoglycemia appear from nowhere
- Avoid processed foods; they are usually sugary, starchy, and high in glycemic index
- Avoid overcooked foods; they promote sugar fluctuations more than raw or lightly cooked foods
- Be careful with breakfast; over-processed breakfast cereals can easily start your day with a sugar swing; use eggs or quark instead

For best results, to achieve better health, not just correct symptoms of hypoglycemia, always choose organic unprocessed produce. These are high in nutrients and low in toxic agricultural residue. They are healthy for you, your family, and the entire planet.

Avoid processed food and food imitations that disguise themselves as food and worse yet health food. Processed food is less nutritious, causes health problems for individuals, and adds garbage to the earth. Long-term studies invariably show that junk eating known also as a standard North American diet is the primary cause behind degenerative decay of humans. We need to finally understand that degenerative diseases are not "caught," "gotten," "or passed on genetically." Their presence simply reflects a cumulative effect of our poor lifestyle and nutritional choices.

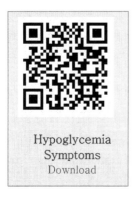

Hypoglycemia
Symptoms
Download

http://goo.gl/dvndpl

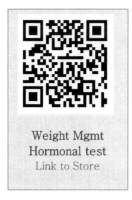

Weight Mgmt
Hormonal test
Link to Store

http://goo.gl/H8505Y

Chapter 36

When good food turns bad

Can good, healthy, fresh, whole, unprocessed food, like a fruit or a vegetable cause unhealthy blood pressure changes? Surprisingly yes, but identifying such can be a bit more complicated than just pointing to a potato or asparagus. There isn't any one food that universally changes blood pressure numbers for everyone. Neither is it true that everyone reacts to foods by reacting with a blood pressure change. Nonetheless, the possibility that food contributes to high or low blood pressure symptoms exists for everyone and it is definitely worth looking into.

It's not food allergy

This chapter is not about food allergy, although severe allergy can cause a blood pressure changes. Everyone knows what food allergy is. One gets hives, diarrhea, or has difficulty breathing. Some people also get skin rashes, cough, or face swelling. Food allergy is usually obvious, because it occurs shortly after ingestion of an allergen. It is also predictable. It always gives the same symptoms after eating the same allergen.

If in doubt one can test a food allergy in a controlled setting. A skin prick session administered by a physician can be quite revealing and point to foods that cause symptoms. Foods that cause body edema should be avoided. You know that, but what you may not know is that body swelling equals a fluid shift, which means a change in blood pressure may follow.

It's not food poisoning

This chapter is not about food poisoning either, which everyone knows what is as well: runs, belly ache, and maybe nausea. On a bad day also major cramps, bloody poop, and a fever. Detecting the source of the misery is not difficult. If shared food also produces shared symptoms it is safe to say that it is food poisoning.

Food poisoning may be tested by analysing a sample of poop for bacteria or parasites. Food poisoning, just like food allergy, can also cause a change in blood pressure. However, food poisoning causes blood pressure change due to fluid *loss* not fluid *shift*.

It's hidden food sensitivity

This chapter is about something different than allergies or food poisoning. It is about food that looks good, smells fresh, and should contribute to health, but yet instead of good health it causes ill-health. I am talking about hidden food sensitivity.

Hidden food sensitivity is not something you may be familiar with. It is not a typical food allergy; it is not food poisoning either, yet food sensitivity can undeniably change how your heart works.

Many people think food reactions are limited to upset stomach and skin rashes, but this is not true. Food sensitivities may contribute or mimic many health predicaments, including blood pressure changes, recurrent infections, or blood sugar fluctuations.

Many ailments, one cause

Dr. Coca has demonstrated that in some instances people can be cured of their chronic ailments by eliminating hidden food sensitivities. Dr. Arthur Fernandez Coca (1875-1959) was a keen observer and a diligent clinician. He wasn't just a medical doctor. He was also a professor, an instructor, a researcher, and a founder of a prominent medical journal.[171] During his cadence as an editor-in-chief he established high standards that put *The Journal of Immunology* in the ranks of peer-reviewed publications, which continues to be is a source of medical discoveries in immunology.

Dr. Coca discovered that food sensitivities can have an amazingly profound effect on the body. They can lead to body-wide inflammation, change in hormone production, and alteration of cardiovascular parameters. Regardless of whether you believe you have or don't have food sensitivities you should take time to test yourself. There is a reason why they are called *hidden*, not obvious, food sensitivities. You simply don't suspect them.

Study the list below. It is a list of conditions that Dr. Coca managed to reverse by detecting and eliminating hidden food sensitivities. Maybe now besides correcting your blood pressure you would be able to eliminate those as well.

- Weight gain, weight loss, weight fluctuations
- Fatigue
- Nervousness, anxiety, depression, irritability
- Dizziness
- Heartburn, indigestion, constipation
- Stomach, intestinal and gallbladder pain
- Colitis, intestinal bleeding, hemorrhoids
- Epilepsy
- Migraines, recurrent headaches
- Nerve pain
- Sinusitis

- Recurrent infections
- Nose bleeds
- Chronic eye inflammation
- Recurrent canker sores
- Diabetes, blood sugar swings
- Hives
- Chest pain, angina, blood pressure fluctuation[172]

But not everyone has health problems due to food sensitivities. Before rushing to suspect food sensitivity behind every ailment you have, first get to know your pulse. People with food sensitivities have an accelerated heart rate, a heart rate that is either fast all day long, or switches between normal slow to rapid, and heart rate changes that cannot be attributed to any emotional or physical challenge.

For example, a heart rate that starts at 68, accelerates to 104 and then decelerates to 74 without an apparent reason looks suspicious. Consider this to be your clue to having a food sensitivity test done. Heart rate in a *healthy* person is remarkably stable. It is not affected by emotions, eating or ordinary movement. Heart rate fluctuations wider than ten beats per minute within a day should alert you to a presence of a significant external stressor, which may happen to be just that… hidden food sensitivity.[173]

After meal napping

Not all cardiovascular inconsistencies are due to food sensitivity. Many people feel sleepy after meals, but that's not because of some sort of allergies, but because of a sudden drop of blood pressure. Tiredness after dinner is common, but it cannot be blamed for a reaction to a specific food. It is a signal that the circulatory system isn't working well.

Digestion is a process that requires a good supply of energy, and that means oxygen. After we eat blood rushes to the digestive organs to deliver oxygen and help with digestion. This causes a temporary "shortage" of blood outside the digestive system. To compensate for this "shortage" blood vessels will narrow. That keeps blood pressure steady and prevents the drop, which in turn prevents a feeling of tiredness.

But the mechanism that steadies blood pressure fails frequently. Studies showed that close to 70% of the elderly in hospitals experience a significant blood pressure drop (at least 20 mmHg systolic) after every single meal.[174] It is all because of circulatory and autonomic nervous system defects.

If you catch yourself napping in the afternoon don't ignore it. Instead, work on restoring failing body circuitry. Start applying all the tips you can recall about supporting autonomic nervous system: better hydration, whole food diet, supplements, blood sugar regulation, cold showers, and exercises. Use whatever you can to add a few more productive hours to your day, every day.

Before the test

Hidden food sensitivities are easy to test and relatively easy to identify from a changing pulse. You don't need any special equipment except for a watch or a stopwatch. There is only one caveat: test may be inaccurate if you are on any heart rate or blood pressure altering medication e.g. blood pressure lowering drugs, anti-depressants anti-histamines, or medication for anxiety.

If you don't know your drugs assume your medication interferes with the test regardless of what you take. Ask your health care provider whether you can temporary suspend your medication or supplementation to be able to perform the test without error-causing factors. If it is not possible to stay medication-free for the time of the test do the test anyhow. If you get some conclusive results, great! Start with those. If you get mixed, inconclusive, or negative results contact a health provider that is familiar with interpretation of the results in challenging situations.

Coca test snapshot

You will need to put aside four consecutive days for the test. Your job is to accurately record the details of your meals as well as correlated heart rate. You will take all measurements while sitting except one in the morning. This one will be done while still lying in bed.

The test will give meaningful results provided you were diligent in recording, did not suffer sunburn or an infection during the time of tests and avoided any heart-straining physical activities. The analysis is simple: if your body perceives a stressor it will accelerate the heart rate over six beats in a minute. An increase of heart rate of ten beats or more after a meal likely pertains to hidden food sensitivity. Repeat the test at different occasions to ensure accuracy and eliminate errors. A heart rate that frequently reaches over 84 beats per minute signifies a very high likelihood that an unsuspected food is stressing your body.

Find the pulse

First, you need to know how to take your pulse. For that you have to be able to find your pulsating artery. The easiest place to locate it is at a wrist or on the neck. To find a pulse on the wrist put your finger just below a bony bump underneath your thumb. Hold it for five to ten seconds. If it pulsates you found it. If it does not you are in a wrong spot. Move your finger slightly and try again.

Alternatively, you can find your pulse on the neck. Your fingers should rest just below the jaw angle. The pulse should appear within three to six seconds. Many people find this spot easier to locate than the one on the wrist.

Once you find the pulsating artery count your heart beats for sixty seconds. Repeat the process several times till you feel confident about your newly acquired skill.

Coca test baselines

Now you are ready to test your baselines. Don't try to skip this step. Without the baselines you won't be able to interpret the results.

There are two baseline checks in the morning. The first one is taken upon waking while still lying in bed. Find your pulse and count your heart rate for sixty seconds, but don't move, uncover, or talk. These will skew the results. Record the number in a log. This is the only time you will be taking heart rate while not-sitting.

Now you can get up and move about, but don't go to the bathroom or eat breakfast yet. You need to record your second baseline before you can do that. Sit down for a minute or two and take your pulse. Record the reading in the log.

For the rest of the day you will be recording details of your meals as well as associated heart rate. The specifics of when and how will be explained a bit later. For now you just need to know to take your third baseline at the end of the day. Sit down and relax for a minute or two just before retiring. Measure your heart rate for sixty seconds and record it, just like the other two baselines in a log.

These three baselines are meal-independent and are meant to reflect your resting heart rate. You will need them to judge the amplitude of your daytime heart accelerations.

Food testing details

Food testing is not very different from testing baselines. All you need to do is to find a pulse and count it for a minute. However, you need to do the count at specific times.

Each meal requires four measurements. These are taken before eating, after eating, a half hour after, and eventually a half hour after that.

You can eat any meals you want, but to make the analysis least complicated stick to one food at a time. It will prevent confusion as to which of the ingredients in the dish is responsible for the positive test. You will get clearer information from eating a carrot alone than eating a carrot cake with seven other ingredients in it.

Copy of use the logs below for recording the data.

Baseline heart rate (HR) numbers:

Day #	Date	HR in bed	HR on waking	HR before bed

Food sensitivity testing

Day #	Time	Food details	HR before food	HR right after	HR ½ hr after food	HR 1 hr after food

The analysis

If you did the test correctly (sitting, relaxed, at required times, with detailed food diary) you should not have any difficulty detecting whether your body is keen on the food you eat. Suspect that a dietary change will do you good if the heart rate goes above eighty-four beats per minute or accelerates more than ten points after a meal.

If the results are unclear, you get different readings for the same food consider other interfering factors. Your body may be responding to anything that you have a contact with from city smog, to toothpaste, to mattress materials, to house dust, to emotional distress. If you are unsure how to proceed seek help of a health practitioner versed in detection of environmental sensitivities and familiar with Coca test.

If you end up with a list of foods that the body reacts to, eliminate them completely from your menu. Continue testing your pulse for any additional deviations. If you managed to lower your pulse and reduce its fluctuations by changing your diet you should notice that many recurrent symptoms may be miraculously going away as well. Keep track of those. You may be amazed how much power you have over your health just by paying attention to your heart.

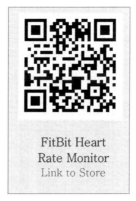

FitBit Heart
Rate Monitor
Link to Store

http://goo.gl/EKC91k

Chapter 37

Off to good health!

By now you may understand that blood pressure numbers can have a much broader diagnostic value than just assessment of a heart muscle. A steady blood pressure and the accompanying steady heart rate is a great gauge of good health. Perfectly adjustable blood pressure is an indicator of a properly functioning nervous system, elasticity of arteries, healthy adrenals as well as agile body reflexes.

Don't discount the numbers displaying on a blood pressure monitor to be used only against hypertensive norms. A blood pressure monitor is one of the greatest health assessment tools every household should have. Blood pressure and heart rate numbers are reliable indicators of body functionality, but only when you know what they mean.

Blood pressure – a hologram of health

Whether normal, high, low, or fluctuating, blood pressure and heart rate are health parameters everyone needs to check regularly. Those with the most stable cardiovascular system are the same individuals who have the greatest ability to adjust to life circumstances and those who cope with stress, whether emotional of physical, the best.

Erratic heart and unpredictable blood pressure swings are indicators of poor health. And although age and genetics can play a role, unless one is more than eight decades old circulatory instability can be attributed more to cumulative lifestyle errors: poor food quality, chronic stress, environmental pollution, overuse of medication, lack of sufficient exercise, lack of fresh air and sunshine, rather than to an unfortunate ancestry line.

Health is a skill, not a pill

When the body ails we are conditioned to think in terms of pharmaceutical help. And sure, medication is the fastest way to bring a temporary relief for racing heart, high blood pressure, and shortness of breath, but it is not, in any way, the best long-term solution for health improvement. You can't strengthen your heart, bring back elasticity to your arteries, restore adrenals, and revive your nervous system with a blood pressure pill.

To have a robust body that is resistant to weakness and degenerative changes you need to build solid health skills. That may not be easy today, because modern health advice is full of controversies and misleading information. Although this book is not meant to teach you health skills, but merely make you understand why your blood pressure behaves in a certain way, you can never go wrong if you follow these guidelines:

- eat more organic vegetables; say no to junk and processed food
- exercise with intent and intensity; put a heart in every move
- enjoy deeper and more harmonious bonds with others, your spouse, kids, co-workers, and other planet inhabitants
- don't hold grudges; shake hands with your enemies; move on
- tickle your photo-responsive cells, bask the morning sun and don't be afraid of natural daylight
- enjoy nature, hike in deep woods, breathe ionized air and rest your eyes on greens
- take off your work boots, high heels, and sandals, touch the earth; it is your home.

Just relax…enjoy the moment. There is no need to rush. Take it step by step towards better health and you will be amazed what's going to happen. You will be on your way to a more robust, zestful, stronger, happier, and all around better you!

DrD

Bigger
picture
YouTube:2:27

https://youtu.be/GOZLvjG5-CA

🍃 *Index*

🦋 *References*

---

[1] MacDougall JD, Tuxen D, Sale DG, Moroz JR, Sutton JR (1985). Arterial blood pressure response to heavy resistance exercise [Abstract]. *J Appl Physiol, 1985 Mar 58(3):785-90* . PMID: 3980383 http://www.ncbi.nlm.nih.gov/pubmed/3980383

[2] McMahon C, Mahmud A, Feely J. (2005). Taking blood pressure - no laughing matter! [Abstract]. *Blood Press Monit. 2005 Apr;10(2):109-10*. PMID: 15812260. http://www.ncbi.nlm.nih.gov/pubmed/15812260

[3] Nemec ED, Mansfield L, Kennedy JW. (1976). Heart rate and blood pressure responses during sexual activity in normal males.[Abstract] *Am Heart J.1976 Sep;92(3):274-7*. PMID: 949020 http://www.ncbi.nlm.nih.gov/pubmed/949020

[4] Drugs that may cause impotence. Retrieved July 24, 2015 from MedlinePlus http://www.nlm.nih.gov/medlineplus/ency/article/004024.htm

[5] Domenic A. Sica (2004). Diuretic-Related Side Effects: Development and Treatment. Retrieved July 24, 2015 from http://www.medscape.com/viewarticle/489521_10

[6] Palatini P1 (1988). Blood pressure behaviour during physical activity [Abstract]. *Sports Med.1988 Jun;5(6):353-74*. PMID: 3041529 http://www.ncbi.nlm.nih.gov/pubmed/3041529

[7] MacDougall JD, Tuxen D, Sale DG, Moroz JR, Sutton JR (1985). Arterial blood pressure response to heavy resistance exercise [Abstract]. *J Appl Physiol, Mar;58(3):785-90* . PMID: 3980383 http://www.ncbi.nlm.nih.gov/pubmed/3980383

[8] Abir-Khalil S, Zaîmi S, Tazi MA, Bendahmane S, Bensaoud O, Benomar M.(2009). Prevalence and predictors of white-coat hypertension in a large database of ambulatory blood pressure monitoring [Abstract]. *East Mediterr Health J. 2009 Mar-Apr;15(2):400-7*. PMID: 19554987 http://www.ncbi.nlm.nih.gov/pubmed/19554987

[9] Gustavsen PH, Høegholm A, Bang LE, Kristensen KS (2003). White coat hypertension is a cardiovascular risk factor: a 10-year follow-up study [Abstract]. *J Hum Hypertens. 2003 Dec;17(12):811-7*. PMID: 14704724 http://www.ncbi.nlm.nih.gov/pubmed/14704724

[10] Farhan Bangash and Rajiv Agarwal (2009). Masked Hypertension and White-Coat Hypertension in Chronic Kidney Disease: A Meta-analysis *Clin J Am Soc Nephrol. 2009 Mar; 4(3): 656–664.* doi: 10.2215/CJN.05391008 PMCID: PMC2653652 http://www.ncbi.nlm.nih.gov/pmc/articles/PMC2653652/

[11] Martin CA1, McGrath BP (2014). White-coat hypertension [Abstract] *Clin Exp Pharmacol Physiol. 2014 Jan;41(1):22-9.* doi: 10.1111/1440-1681.12114 PMID: 23682974 http://www.ncbi.nlm.nih.gov/pubmed/23682974

[12] Hypertension Canada (2014). *Diagnosis, 2014 CHEP Recommendations.* Retrieved May 22, 2015 from https://www.hypertension.ca/en/professional/chep/diagnosis-measurement/criteria-for-diagnosis-a-recommendations-for-follow-up

[13] Elisabete Pinto (2007). Blood pressure and ageing. *Postgrad Med J. 2007 Feb; 83(976): 109–114.* doi: 10.1136/pgmj.2006.048371 PMCID: PMC2805932 http://www.ncbi.nlm.nih.gov/pmc/articles/PMC2805932/

[14] Perlmuter LC1, Sarda G, Casavant V, Mosnaim AD(2013). A review of the etiology, associated comorbidities, and treatment of orthostatic hypotension [Abstract]. *Am J Ther. 2013 May-Jun;20(3):279-91.* doi: 10.1097/MJT.0b013e31828bfb7f. PMID: 23656967 http://www.ncbi.nlm.nih.gov/pubmed/23656967

[15] Bjørn Hildrum, Arnstein Mykletun, Eystein Stordal, Ingvar Bjelland, Alv A Dahl, and Jostein Holmen (2007). Association of low blood pressure with anxiety and depression: the Nord-Trøndelag Health Study. *J Epidemiol & Community Health. 2007 Jan; 61(1): 53–58.* doi: 10.1136/jech.2005.044966 PMCID: PMC2465598 http://www.ncbi.nlm.nih.gov/pmc/articles/PMC2465598/

[16] Rita Moretti, Paola Torre, Rodolfo M Antonello, Davide Manganaro, Cristina Vilotti, and Gilberto Pizzolato (2008). Risk factors for vascular dementia: Hypotension as a key point. *Vasc Health Risk Manag. 2008 Apr; 4(2): 395–402.* PMCID: PMC2496988 http://www.ncbi.nlm.nih.gov/pmc/articles/PMC2496988/

[17] Charlson ME, de Moraes CG, Link A, Wells MT, Harmon G, Peterson JC, Ritch R, Liebmann JM (2014). Nocturnal systemic hypotension increases the risk of glaucoma progression [Abstract]. *Ophthalmology. 2014 Oct;121(10):2004-12.* doi: 10.1016/j.ophtha.2014.04.016. PMID: 24869467 http://www.ncbi.nlm.nih.gov/pubmed/24869467

[18] Pirodda A1, Ferri GG, Modugno GC, Gaddi A. (1999). Hypotension and sensorineural hearing loss: a possible correlation [Abstract]. *Acta Otolaryngol 1999;119(7):758-62.* PMID: 10687931 http://www.ncbi.nlm.nih.gov/pubmed/10687931

[19] Arai M1, Takada T, Nozue M. (2003). Orthostatic tinnitus: an otological presentation of spontaneous intracranial hypotension [Abstract]. *Auris Nasus Larynx. 2003 Feb;30(1):85-7.* PMID: 12589857 http://www.ncbi.nlm.nih.gov/pubmed/12589857

[20] Isildak H, Albayram S, Isildak (2010). Spontaneous intracranial hypotension syndrome accompanied by bilateral hearing loss and venous engorgement in the internal acoustic canal and positional change of audiography [Abstract]. *H.J Craniofac Surg. 2010 Jan;21(1):165-7.* doi: 10.1097/SCS.0b013e3181c50e11 PMID: 20072012 http://www.ncbi.nlm.nih.gov/pubmed/20072012

[21] Jean-Louis Vincent and Diego Castanares Zapatero (2008).The role of hypotension in the development of acute renal failure. *Oxford JournalsMedicine & Health Nephrology Dialysis Transplantation, 24 (2) p. 337-338.*
http://ndt.oxfordjournals.org/content/24/2/337.full

[22] Fanaroff AA1, Fanaroff JM.(2006). Short- and long-term consequences of hypotension in ELBW infants [Abstract]. *Semin Perinatol. 2006 Jun;30(3):151-5.* PMID: 16813974
http://www.ncbi.nlm.nih.gov/pubmed/16813974

[23] Robert D Langer, Theodore G Ganiats, Elizabeth Barrett-Connor (1989). Paradoxical survival of elderly men with high blood pressure. *BMJ, 298, p.1356-1357.*
http://www.ncbi.nlm.nih.gov/pmc/articles/PMC1836610/pdf/bmj00232-0032.pdf

[24] June Liu (2011). Correlation Among Different Variables and Life Expectancy. *Undergraduate Journal of Mathematical Modeling: One + Two, 3(2) art.2.*
http://scholarcommons.usf.edu/cgi/viewcontent.cgi?article=4820&context=ujmm

[25] Michael Schachter (2004). Diurnal Rhythms, the Renin-Angiotensin System and Antihypertensive Therapy. *British Journal of Cardiology, 2004;11(4).*
http://www.medscape.com/viewarticle/490535_2

[26] Silva AP1, Moreira C, Bicho M, Paiva T, Clara JG. (2000). Nocturnal sleep quality and circadian blood pressure variation [Abstract]. *Rev Port Cardiol [Abstract]. 2000 Oct;19(10):991-1005.* PMID: 11126112
http://www.ncbi.nlm.nih.gov/pubmed/11126112

[27] Michael Schachter (2004). Diurnal Rhythms, the Renin-Angiotensin System and Antihypertensive Therapy. *British Journal of Cardiology, 2004;11(4).*
http://www.medscape.com/viewarticle/490535_2

[28] A.M. Birkenhäger, A.H. van den Meiracker (2007). Causes and consequences of a non-dipping blood pressure profile. *The Netherlands Journal of Medicine, April 2007 64(4) p. 127-131.* http://njmonline.nl/getpdf.php?id=518

[29] Barksdale DJ, Woods-Giscombé C, Logan JG Stress, cortisol, and nighttime blood pressure dipping in nonhypertensive Black American women [Abstract]. *Biol Res Nurs. 2013 Jul;15(3):330-7.* doi: 0.1177/1099800411433291 PMID: 22472903
http://www.ncbi.nlm.nih.gov/pubmed/22472903

[30] Health Stats. 24-hr ABPM Patterns. Retrieved May 22, 2015 from
http://www.healthstats.com/index3.php?page=bp-abpm-24hrabpm-pattern

[31] B. Bouhanick, V. Bongard, J. Amar, S. Bousquel, B. Chamontin (2008). Prognostic value of nocturnal blood pressure and reverse-dipping status on the occurrence of cardiovascular events in hypertensive diabetic patients. *Diabetes & Metabolism Dec 2008 34(6) p. 560-567.* doi : 10.1016/j.diabet.2008.05.005 http://www.em-consulte.com/en/article/195988

[32] Fagard RH (2009). Dipping pattern of nocturnal blood pressure in patients with hypertension [Abstract}. *Expert Rev Cardiovasc Ther. 2009 Jun;7(6):599-605.* doi: 10.1586/erc.09.35. PMID: 19505275 http://www.ncbi.nlm.nih.gov/pubmed/19505275

[33] Fagard RH (2009). Dipping pattern of nocturnal blood pressure in patients with hypertension. *Expert Rev Cardiovasc Ther. 2009 Jun;7(6):599-605.*
http://www.medscape.com/viewarticle/705780

[34] Tan Xu MM, Yong-Qing Zhang MBBS andXue-Rui Tan MD (2012). The Dilemma of Nocturnal Blood Pressure. The *Journal of Clinical Hypertension. 14(11), p. 787–791, November 2012.* DOI: 10.1111/jch.12003 http://onlinelibrary.wiley.com/doi/10.1111/jch.12003/full

[35] Kazuomi Kario, Thomas G. Pickering, Takefumi Matsuo, Satoshi Hoshide, Joseph E. Schwartz, Kazuyuki Shimada (2001). Stroke Prognosis and Abnormal Nocturnal Blood Pressure Falls in Older Hypertensives. *Am Heart Assoc, Scientific Contributions, March 21, 2001.* http://hyper.ahajournals.org/content/38/4/852.full

[36] Thomas G. Pickering MD, DPhil (2008). Ambulatory Blood Pressure and Diseases of the Eye: Can Low Nocturnal Blood Pressure Be Harmful? *The Journal of Clinical Hypertension 10(5), p. 411–414, May 2008.* DOI: 10.1111/j.1751-7176.2008.08048.x http://onlinelibrary.wiley.com/doi/10.1111/j.1751-7176.2008.08048.x/full

[37] Kelli Gibson, Robert Lee Page II (2007). What's Up with Morning Blood Pressure? *Pharmacy Times, June 1, 2007.* Retrieved May 24, 2015 from http://www.pharmacytimes.com/p2p/2007-06-6594

[38] Lin-Fang Chen, Ju-Chi Liu, Mei-Yeh Wang, Shiow-Li Hwang, Pei-Shan Tsai (2011). Extreme Nocturnal Blood Pressure Dipping is Associated With Increased Arterial Stiffness in Individuals With Components of the Metabolic Syndrome. *Journal of Experimental & Clinical Medicine 3(3) p.132–136 June 2011.* doi:10.1016/j.jecm.2011.04.007 http://www.sciencedirect.com/science/article/pii/S1878331711000635

[39] J. Hope, (2013). 90% of Britons don't know their blood pressure rate - and more than five million are unaware they have potentially fatal condition. Retrieved July 28, 2015 from DailyMail http://www.dailymail.co.uk/news/article-2421435/90-Britons-dont-know-blood-pressure-rate--million-unaware-potentially-fatal-condition.html

[40] M.E.Dallas (2015). Half of People With High BP Don't Know It. Retrieved July 28, 2015 from WebMD. http://www.webmd.com/hypertension-high-blood-pressure/news/20130903/half-of-people-with-high-blood-pressure-dont-know-it

[41] Chapotot F, Gronfier C, Jouny C, Muzet A, Brandenberger G.(1998). Cortisol secretion is related to electroencephalographic alertness in human subjects during daytime wakefulness [Abstract]. *J Clin Endocrinol Metab. 1998 Dec;83(12):4263-8.* PMID: 9851761 http://www.ncbi.nlm.nih.gov/pubmed/9851761

[42] Cortisol awakening response. Wikipedia. Retrieved May 24, 2015 from http://en.wikipedia.org/wiki/Cortisol_awakening_response

[43] Kelli Gibson, Robert Lee Page II (2007). What's Up with Morning Blood Pressure? *Pharmacy Times, June 1, 2007.* Retrieved May 24, 2015 from http://www.pharmacytimes.com/p2p/2007-06-6594

[44] Kelli Gibson, Robert Lee Page II (2007). What's Up with Morning Blood Pressure? *Pharmacy Times, June 1, 2007.* Retrieved May 24, 2015 from http://www.pharmacytimes.com/p2p/2007-06-6594

[45] Kazuomi Kario (2010). Morning Surge in Blood Pressure and Cardiovascular Risk, Evidence and Perspectives . *Hypertension, Brief Reviews Sept 7, 2007.* http://hyper.ahajournals.org/content/56/5/765.full

[46] Stephen Sinatra (2014). High Blood Pressure Readings in the Morning. Retrieved May 24, 2015 from http://www.drsinatra.com/high-blood-pressure-readings-in-the-morning

[47] Stephen Sinatra (2014). High Blood Pressure Readings in the Morning. Retrieved May 24, 2015 from http://www.drsinatra.com/high-blood-pressure-readings-in-the-morning

[48] Kelli Gibson, Robert Lee Page II (2007). What's Up with Morning Blood Pressure? *Pharmacy Times, June 1, 2007.* Retrieved May 24, 2015 from http://www.pharmacytimes.com/p2p/2007-06-6594

[49] Kazuomi Kario (2005). Morning hypertension: a pitfall of current hypertensive management. *JMAJ 48(5) 234-240, 2005.* http://www.med.or.jp/english/pdf/2005_05/234_240.pdf

[50] Addison`s disease. Wikipedia. Retrieved May 26, 2015 from http://en.wikipedia.org/wiki/Addison's_disease

[51] Criqui MH, Langer RD, Reed DM (1989). Dietary alcohol, calcium, and potassium. Independent and combined effects on blood pressure [Abstract]. *Circulation. 1989 Sep;80(3):609-14.* PMID: 2766513 http://www.ncbi.nlm.nih.gov/pubmed/2766513

[52] Terry R. Hartley, Bong Hee Sung, Gwendolyn A. Pincomb, Thomas L. Whitsett, Michael F. Wilson, William R. Lovallo (2000). Hypertension Risk Status and Effect of Caffeine on Blood Pressure. *Hypertension, Scientific Contributions, Jan 27, 2000.* http://hyper.ahajournals.org/content/36/1/137.long [Abstract] http://www.ncbi.nlm.nih.gov/pubmed/10904026

[53] James, Jack E. (2004). Critical Review of Dietary Caffeine and Blood Pressure: A Relationship That Should Be Taken More Seriously [Abstract]. *Psychosomatic Medicine: January/February 2004 – 66(1) pp 63-71.* http://www.psychosomaticmedicine.org/content/66/1/63.full.pdf+html

[54] Youngmok Kima, Kevin L. Goodnera, Jong-Dae Parkb, Jeong Choib, Stephen T. Talcott (2011). Changes in antioxidant phytochemicals and volatile composition of Camellia sinensis by oxidation during tea fermentation [Abstract]. *Food Chemistry 129(4), 1331–1342, 15 December 2011.* http://www.sciencedirect.com/science/article/pii/S0308814611007011

[55] Hodgson JM, Puddey IB, Burke V, Beilin LJ, Jordan N (1999). Effects on blood pressure of drinking green and black tea. *J Hypertens. 1999 Apr;17(4):457-63.* PMID: 10404946 .http://www.ncbi.nlm.nih.gov/pubmed/10404946

[56] Lenny R. Vartanian, PhD, Marlene B. Schwartz, PhD, and Kelly D. Brownell, PhD (2007). Effects of Soft Drink Consumption on Nutrition and Health: A Systematic Review and Meta-Analysis. *Am J Public Health. 2007 April; 97(4): 667–675.* doi: 10.2105/AJPH.2005.083782 PMCID: PMC1829363 http://www.ncbi.nlm.nih.gov/pmc/articles/PMC1829363

[57] H E de Wardener, G A MacGregor (2002). Harmful effects of dietary salt in addition to hypertension. *Journal of Human Hypertension, April 2002, 16(4) pp 213-223* http://www.nature.com/jhh/journal/v16/n4/full/1001374a.html

[58] Stephen Daniells (2010). Salt's harmful effects may extend to artery hardening. *Food navigator 19-Feb-2010.* Retrieved June 2, 2015 from http://www.foodnavigator.com/Science/Salt-s-harmful-effects-may-extend-to-artery-hardening

[59] Salt Shockers Slideshow: High-Sodium Surprises (Feb 4, 2014). Retrieved June 2, 1015 from http://www.webmd.com/diet/ss/slideshow-salt-shockers

[60] Ian J Brown, Ioanna Tzoulaki, Vanessa Candeias and Paul Elliott (2009). Salt intakes around the world: implications for public health. *International Journal of Epidemiology 38(3) pp. 791-813*. http://ije.oxfordjournals.org/content/38/3/791.full

[61] Mara Betsch. 25 Surprisingly Salty Processed Foods. Retrieved June 2, 2015 from http://www.health.com/health/gallery/0,,20365078,00.html

[62] Ian J Brown, Ioanna Tzoulaki, Vanessa Candeias and Paul Elliott (2009). Salt intakes around the world: implications for public health. *International Journal of Epidemiology 38(3) pp. 791-813*. http://ije.oxfordjournals.org/content/38/3/791.full

[63] Sodium (Na) in Blood (September 04, 2012). Retrieved June 9, 2015 from http://www.webmd.com/a-to-z-guides/sodium-na-in-blood

[64] Low Sodium Diet. Wikipedia. Retrieved June 9, 2015 from http://en.wikipedia.org/wiki/Low_sodium_diet

[65] Michelle Robida (2006). No Difference in the Effectiveness of Albumin Versus Normal Saline for the Treatment of Hypotension in Mechanically Ventilated Preterm Infants. Retrieved June 9, 2015 from University of Michigan Department of Pediatrics Evidence-Based Pediatrics Web Site http://www.med.umich.edu/pediatrics/ebm/cats/albumin2.htm

[66] Greg A. Knoll, Jenny A. Grabowski, Geoffrey F. Dervin and Keith O'Rourke (2003). A Randomized, Controlled Trial of Albumin versus Saline for the Treatment of Intradialytic Hypotension. *Journal of the American Society of Nephrology Nov 12, 2003*. http://jasn.asnjournals.org/content/15/2/487.full

[67] Graham P Bates and Veronica S Miller (2008). Sweat rate and sodium loss during work in the heat. *J Occup Med Toxicol. 2008; 3: 4*. doi: 10.1186/1745-6673-3-4 PMCID: PMC2267797 http://www.ncbi.nlm.nih.gov/pmc/articles/PMC2267797/

[68] Graham P Bates and Veronica S Miller (2008). Sweat rate and sodium loss during work in the heat. *J Occup Med Toxicol. 2008; 3: 4*. doi: 10.1186/1745-6673-3-4 PMCID: PMC2267797 http://www.ncbi.nlm.nih.gov/pmc/articles/PMC2267797/

[69] Sodium. Ministry of Health, Nutrient reference values for Australia and News Zealand. Retreived June 9, 2015 from https://www.nrv.gov.au/nutrients/sodium

[70] Annie B. Bond (2008). 13 Symptoms of Chronic Dehydration (June 7, 2008). Retrieved June 14, 2015 from http://www.care2.com/greenliving/13-symptoms-of-chronic-dehydration.html

[71] Isaac Eliaz (2012). Are You Chronically Dehydrated? (August 1, 2012). Retrieved June 14, 2015 from http://www.rodalenews.com/chronic-dehydration

[72] Dehydration. Wikipedia. Retrieved June 14, 2015 from http://en.wikipedia.org/wiki/Dehydration

[73] Dehydration. Mayo Clinic, Diseases and Conditions, Complications, (Feb 12, 2014). Retrieved June 16, 2015 from http://www.mayoclinic.org/diseases-conditions/dehydration/basics/complications/con-20030056

[74] Stephen Daniells (2010). Salt's harmful effects may extend to artery hardening. Food navigator 19-Feb-2010. Retrieved June 2, 2015 from http://www.foodnavigator.com/Science/Salt-s-harmful-effects-may-extend-to-artery-hardening

[75] Merck Manual, Consumer Version. Overview of disorders of fluid volume. Retrieved June 23, 2015 from https://www.merckmanuals.com/home/SearchResults?query=Overview+of+Disorders+of+Fluid+Volume

[76] Jean W H Yong (2009). The Chemical Composition and Biological Properties of Coconut (Cocos nucifera L.) Water. *Molecules 2009, 14(12), 5144-5164.* doi:10.3390/molecules14125144

[77] Coconut water. Wikipedia. Retrieved June 9, 2015 from http://en.wikipedia.org/wiki/Coconut_water

[78] Campbell-Falck D, Thomas T, Falck TM, Tutuo N, Clem K (2000). The intravenous use of coconut water [Abstract]. *Am J Emerg Med. 2000 Jan;18(1):108-11.* PMID: 10674546 .http://www.ncbi.nlm.nih.gov/pubmed/10674546

[79] Karl S. Kruszelnicki (2015). Retrieved from ABC Science on July 20, 2015. http://www.abc.net.au/science/articles/2014/12/09/4143229.htm

[80] Jean W H Yong (2009). The Chemical Composition and Biological Properties of Coconut (Cocos nucifera L.) Water. *Molecules 2009, 14(12), 5144-5164.* doi:10.3390/molecules14125144

[81] Njelekela M, Sato T, Nara Y, Miki T, Kuga S, Noguchi T, Kanda T, Yamori M, Ntogwisangu J, Masesa Z, Mashalla Y, Mtabaji J, Yamori Y. (2003) Nutritional variation and cardiovascular risk factors in Tanzania--rural-urban difference [Abstract]. *S Afr Med J. 2003 Apr;93(4):295-9.* PMID: 12806724 http://www.ncbi.nlm.nih.gov/pubmed/12806724

[82] Circadian Rhythm, Wikipedia. Retrieved June 23, 2015 from https://en.wikipedia.org/wiki/Circadian_rhythm

[83] Ibid https://en.wikipedia.org/wiki/Circadian_rhythm

[84] Ibid https://en.wikipedia.org/wiki/Circadian_rhythm

[85] Redon J (2004). The normal circadian pattern of blood pressure: implications for treatment [Abstract]. *Int J Clin Pract Suppl. 2004 Dec;(145):3-8.* PMID: 15617452 http://www.ncbi.nlm.nih.gov/pubmed/15617452

[86] Crivaldo Gomes Cardoso, Jr, Ricardo Saraceni Gomides, Andréia Cristiane Carrenho Queiroz, Luiz Gustavo Pinto, Fernando da Silveira Lobo, Tais Tinucci, Décio Mion, Jr, and Claudia Lucia de Moraes (2010). Acute and Chronic Effects of Aerobic and Resistance Exercise on Ambulatory Blood Pressure. *Clinics (Sao Paulo). 2010 Mar; 65(3): 317–325.* doi: 10.1590/S1807-59322010000300013 PMC2845774 http://www.ncbi.nlm.nih.gov/pmc/articles/PMC2845774/

[87] Narloch JA, Brandstater ME (1995). Influence of breathing technique on arterial blood pressure during heavy weight lifting [Abstract}. *Arch Phys Med Rehabil. 1995 May;76(5):457-62.* PMID: 7741618 http://www.ncbi.nlm.nih.gov/pubmed/7741618

[88] West DJ, Cook CJ, Beaven MC, Kilduff LP (2014). *J Strength Cond Res. 2014 Jun;28(6):1524-8.* The influence of the time of day on core temperature and lower body power output in elite rugby union sevens players. PMID: 24149752 .http://www.ncbi.nlm.nih.gov/pubmed/24149752

[89] Hydrotherapy Wikipedia. Retrieved 23 June 2015 from https://en.wikipedia.org/wiki/Hydrotherapy

[90] Hydrotherapy information (Sep 20, 2008). Natural Therapy Pages. Retrieved June 23, 2015 from http://www.naturaltherapypages.com.au/article/hydrotherapy

[91] A Mooventhan and L Nivethitha (2014). Scientific Evidence-Based Effects of Hydrotherapy on Various Systems of the Body. *N Am J Med Sci. 2014 May; 6(5): 199–209*. doi: 10.4103/1947-2714.132935 PMC4049052 http://www.ncbi.nlm.nih.gov/pmc/articles/PMC4049052/

[92] Ibid http://www.ncbi.nlm.nih.gov/pmc/articles/PMC4049052/

[93] Brown adipose tissue, Wikipedia. Retrieved 23 June 2015 from https://en.wikipedia.org/wiki/Brown_adipose_tissue

[94] Den Hond E, Celis H, Vandenhoven G, O'Brien E, Staessen JA (2003). Determinants of white-coat syndrome assessed by ambulatory blood pressure or self-measured home blood pressure [Abstract]. *Blood Press Monit. 2003 Feb;8(1):37-40*. PMID: 12604935 http://www.ncbi.nlm.nih.gov/pubmed/12604935

[95] Lizette Borreli (June 24, 2014). Benefits of Cold Showers: 7 Reasons Why Taking Cool Showers Is Good For Your Health. Retrieved June 23, 2015 from Medical Daily http://www.medicaldaily.com/benefits-cold-showers-7-reasons-why-taking-cool-showers-good-your-health-289524

[96] Aaron M. Cypess, M.D., Ph.D., M.M.Sc., Sanaz Lehman, M.B., B.S., Gethin Williams, M.B., B.S., Ph.D., Ilan Tal, Ph.D., Dean Rodman, M.D., Allison B. Goldfine, M.D., Frank C. Kuo, M.D., Ph.D., Edwin L. Palmer, M.D., Yu-Hua Tseng, Ph.D., Alessandro Doria, M.D., Ph.D., M.P.H., Gerald M. Kolodny, M.D., and C. Ronald Kahn, M.D. (2009). Identification and Importance of Brown Adipose Tissue in Adult Humans. *N Engl J Med 2009; 360:1509-1517 April 9, 2009* doi: 10.1056/NEJMoa0810780 http://www.nejm.org/doi/full/10.1056/NEJMoa0810780

[97] A Mooventhan and L Nivethitha (2014). Scientific Evidence-Based Effects of Hydrotherapy on Various Systems of the Body. *N Am J Med Sci. 2014 May; 6(5): 199–209*. doi: 10.4103/1947-2714.132935 PMC4049052 http://www.ncbi.nlm.nih.gov/pmc/articles/PMC4049052/

[98] Jens Jordan, MD; John R. Shannon, MD; Bonnie K. Black, BSN; Yasmine Ali, BS; Mary Farley; Fernando Costa, MD; Andre Diedrich, MD; Rose Marie Robertson, MD; Italo Biaggioni, MD; David Robertson, MD (1999). The Pressor Response to Water Drinking in Humans, A Sympathetic Reflex? *Circulation, Clinical Investigation and Reports, Sept 15, 1999*. Retrieved June 28, 2015 from http://circ.ahajournals.org/content/101/5/504.full

[99] Leigh MacMillan (2010). Plain water has surprising impact on blood pressure. Reporter, Vanderbilt University Medical Center's Weekly Newspaper. Retrieved 23 June 2015 from http://www.mc.vanderbilt.edu:8080/reporter/index.html?ID=9047

[100] Ibid http://circ.ahajournals.org/content/101/5/504.full

[101] Julian M Stewart (2015). Orthostatic Intolerance (Feb, 02, 2015). Retrieved June 28, 2015 from Medscape http://emedicine.medscape.com/article/902155-overview

[102] Lyall A. J. Higginson (2014). Orthostatic Hypotension, Merck Manual, Professional Version. Retrieved June 28, 2015 from http://www.merckmanuals.com/professional/cardiovascular-disorders/symptoms-of-cardiovascular-disorders/orthostatic-hypotension

[103] Ar Kar Aung, Susan J. Corcoran, Vathy Nagalingam, Eldho Paul, and Harvey H. Newnham (2012). Prevalence, Associations, and Risk Factors for Orthostatic Hypotension in Medical, Surgical, and Trauma Inpatients: An Observational Cohort Study. *Ochsner J. 2012 Spring; 12(1): 35–41.* PMC3307503
http://www.ncbi.nlm.nih.gov/pmc/articles/PMC3307503/

[104] Low PA (2008). Prevalence of orthostatic hypotension. *Clin Auton Res. 2008 Mar;18 Suppl 1:8-13.* doi: 10.1007/s10286-007-1001-3. PMID: 18368301
http://www.ncbi.nlm.nih.gov/pubmed/18368301

[105] Juan J. Figueroa, Jeffrey R. Basford, and Philip A. Low (2008). Preventing and treating orthostatic hypotension: As easy as A, B, C. Cleve *Clin J Med. 2010 May; 77(5): 298–306.* doi: 10.3949/ccjm.77a.09118 PMC2888469
http://www.ncbi.nlm.nih.gov/pmc/articles/PMC2888469/

[106] Low PA (2008). Prevalence of orthostatic hypotension. *Clin Auton Res. 2008 Mar;18 Suppl 1:8-13.* doi: 10.1007/s10286-007-1001-3. PMID: 18368301
http://www.ncbi.nlm.nih.gov/pubmed/18368301

[107] Ibid http://www.ncbi.nlm.nih.gov/pubmed/18368301

[108] Ibid http://www.ncbi.nlm.nih.gov/pubmed/18368301

[109] Ooi WL1, Hossain M, Lipsitz LA (2000). The association between orthostatic hypotension and recurrent falls in nursing home residents [Abstract]. *Am J Med. 2000 Feb;108(2):106-11.* PMID: 11126303 http://www.ncbi.nlm.nih.gov/pubmed/11126303

[110] Angelousi A1, Girerd N, Benetos A, Frimat L, Gautier S, Weryha G, Boivin JM (2014). Association between orthostatic hypotension and cardiovascular risk, cerebrovascular risk, cognitive decline and falls as well as overall mortality: a systematic review and meta-analysis. *J Hypertens. 2014 Aug;32(8):1562-71; discussion 1571.* doi: 10.1097/HJH.0000000000000235 PMID: 24879490
http://www.ncbi.nlm.nih.gov/pubmed/24879490

[111] Low PA (2008). Prevalence of orthostatic hypotension. *Clin Auton Res. 2008 Mar;18 Suppl 1:8-13.* doi: 10.1007/s10286-007-1001-3. PMID: 18368301
http://www.ncbi.nlm.nih.gov/pubmed/18368301

[112] European Society of Cardiology (2009). Guidelines for the diagnosis and management of syncope (version 2009). *European Heart Journal. pp 2631-2671*
doi:http://dx.doi.org/10.1093/eurheartj/ehp298

[113] Juan J. Figueroa, Jeffrey R. Basford, and Philip A. Low (2008). Preventing and treating orthostatic hypotension: As easy as A, B, C. Cleve *Clin J Med. 2010 May; 77(5): 298–306.* doi: 10.3949/ccjm.77a.09118 PMC2888469
http://www.ncbi.nlm.nih.gov/pmc/articles/PMC2888469/

[114] Ibid http://www.ncbi.nlm.nih.gov/pmc/articles/PMC2888469/

[115] Micturition syncope. Wikipedia. Retrieved August 9, 2015 from
https://en.wikipedia.org/wiki/Micturition_syncope

[116] Guidelines for the diagnosis and management of syncope (2009). *European Heart Journal (2009) 30, 2631–2671.* doi:10.1093/eurheartj/ehp298
http://eurheartj.oxfordjournals.org/content/ehj/30/21/2631.full.pdf

[117] European Society of Cardiology (2009). Guidelines for the diagnosis and management of syncope (version 2009). *European Heart Journal. pp 2631-2671* doi:http://dx.doi.org/10.1093/eurheartj/ehp298

[118] Gibbons CH, Freeman R. (2006). Delayed orthostatic hypotension: a frequent cause of orthostatic intolerance [Abstract]. *Neurology. 2006 Jul 11;67(1):28-32.* PMID: 16832073 http://www.ncbi.nlm.nih.gov/pubmed/16832073

[119] Michael J. Reichgott (1990). Clinical Methods: The History, Physical, and Laboratory Examinations, 3rd edition, Ch 76 Clinical Evidence of Dysautonomia. http://www.ncbi.nlm.nih.gov/books/NBK400/

[120] Lonsdale D, Shamberger RJ, Obrenovich ME. (2011). Exaggerated Autonomic Asymmetry: A Clue to Nutrient Deficiency Dysautonomia. *WebmedCentral Alternative Medicine 2011;2(4):WMC001854* doi: 10.9754/journal.wmc.2011.001854 http://www.webmedcentral.com/article_view/1854

[121] Derrick Lonsdale (2009). Dysautonomia, A Heuristic Approach to a Revised Model for Etiology of Disease. *Evid Based Complement Alternat Med. 2009 Mar; 6(1): 3–10.* doi: 10.1093/ecam/nem064 PMC2644268 http://www.ncbi.nlm.nih.gov/pmc/articles/PMC2644268/

[122] Lonsdale D, Shamberger RJ, Obrenovich ME. (2011). Exaggerated Autonomic Asymmetry: A Clue to Nutrient Deficiency Dysautonomia. *WebmedCentral Alternative Medicine 2011;2(4):WMC001854* doi: 10.9754/journal.wmc.2011.001854 http://www.webmedcentral.com/article_view/1854

[123] Ibid http://www.webmedcentral.com/article_view/1854

[124] Beriberi, Wikipedia. Retrieved June 28, 2015 from https://en.wikipedia.org/?title=Beriberi

[125] Mercola (2009). Warning: Potentially Life Threatening Vitamin Deficiency Affects 25% of Adults Retreived June 28, 2015 from http://articles.mercola.com/sites/articles/archive/2009/05/19/warning-potentially-life-threatening-vitamin-deficiency-affects-25-percent-of-adults.aspx

[126] Government of Canada, Statistics Canada. Vitamin B12 status of Canadians, 2009 to 2011. Retrieved June 28, 2015 from http://www.statcan.gc.ca/pub/82-625-x/2012001/article/11731-eng.htm

[127] Langley WF, Mann D (1991). Central nervous system magnesium deficiency. *Arch Intern Med. 1991 Mar;151(3):593-6.* PMID: 2001142 http://www.ncbi.nlm.nih.gov/pubmed/2001142

[128] Leo D. Galland, Sidney M. Baker, Robert K McLellan. Magnesium Deficiency in the Pathogenesis of Mitral Valve Prolapse. Retrieved June 28, 2015 from http://www.mdheal.org/magnesiu.htm

[129] Mark Sircus (2009, December 8). Magnesium in Neurological Diseases and Emotions. Retrieved June 28, 2015 from http://drsircus.com/medicine/magnesium/magnesium-in-neurological-diseases-and-emotions

[130] Enrivomedica. Ancient Minerals,The Bad News about Magnesium Food Sources. Retrieved June 28, 2015 from http://www.ancient-minerals.com/magnesium-sources/dietary/

[131] Ibid http://www.ancient-minerals.com/magnesium-sources/dietary/

[132] Enrivomedica. Ancient Minerals, Need More Magnesium? 10 Signs to Watch For. Retrieved June 28, 2015 from http://www.ancient-minerals.com/magnesium-deficiency/need-more/

[133] A Mooventhan and L Nivethitha (2014). Scientific Evidence-Based Effects of Hydrotherapy on Various Systems of the Body. *N Am J Med Sci. 2014 May; 6(5): 199–209.* doi: 10.4103/1947-2714.132935 PMC4049052 http://www.ncbi.nlm.nih.gov/pmc/articles/PMC4049052/

[134] Ibid http://www.ncbi.nlm.nih.gov/pmc/articles/PMC4049052/

[135] Ibid http://www.ncbi.nlm.nih.gov/pmc/articles/PMC4049052/

[136] Ibid http://www.ncbi.nlm.nih.gov/pmc/articles/PMC4049052/

[137] Norephinephrine, Wikipedia. Retrieved June 28, 2015 from https://en.wikipedia.org/wiki/Norepinephrine

[138] Norephinephrine, Drugs.com Retrieved June 28, 2015 from http://www.drugs.com/mtm/norepinephrine.html

[139] Julian M. Stewart, MD, PhD (2013). Common Syndromes of Orthostatic Intolerance. *Pediatrics. 2013 May; 131(5): 968–980.* PMCID: PMC3639459 doi: 10.1542/peds.2012-2610 http://www.ncbi.nlm.nih.gov/pmc/articles/PMC3639459

[140] Dr. Bryan P. Walsh. The Adrenal Glands. Retrieved August 12, 2015 from Precision Nutrition http://www.precisionnutrition.com/what-do-the-adrenal-glands-do

[141] Orthostatic Hypertension, Wikipedia. Retrieved June 28, 2015 from https://en.wikipedia.org/wiki/Orthostatic_hypertension

[142] Dr. Bryan P. Walsh. The Adrenal Glands. Retrieved August 12, 2015 from Precision Nutrition http://www.precisionnutrition.com/what-do-the-adrenal-glands-do

[143] Ferrari E, Cravello L, Falvo F, Barili L, Solerte SB, Fioravanti M, Magri F. (2008). Neuroendocrine features in extreme longevity [Abstract]. *Exp Gerontol. 2008 Feb;43(2):88-94.* PMID: 17764865 http://www.ncbi.nlm.nih.gov/pubmed/17764865

[144] Blevins JK, Coxworth JE, Herndon JG, Hawkes K (2013). Brief communication: Adrenal androgens and aging: Female chimpanzees (Pan troglodytes) compared with women. *Am J Phys Anthropol. 2013 Aug;151(4):643-8.* doi: 10.1002/ajpa.22300. PMID: 23818143 http://www.ncbi.nlm.nih.gov/pubmed/23818143

[145] Traish AM, Kang HP, Saad F, Guay AT (2011). Dehydroepiandrosterone (DHEA)--a precursor steroid or an active hormone in human physiology..*J Sex Med. 2011 Nov;8(11):2960-82*; PMID: 22032408 doi: 10.1111/j.1743-6109.2011.02523.x. http://www.ncbi.nlm.nih.gov/pubmed/22032408

[146] Stress Management for Health Course. Stress and the Role of Breathing. Retrieved June 28, 2015 from http://stresscourse.tripod.com/id20.html

[147] Lundberg JO (2008). Nitric oxide and the paranasal sinuses [Abstract]. *Anat Rec (Hoboken). 2008 Nov;291(11):1479-84.* doi: 10.1002/ar.20782. PMID: 18951492 http://www.ncbi.nlm.nih.gov/pubmed/18951492

[148] Biological function of nitric oxide, Wikipedia. Retrieved June 28, 2015 from https://en.wikipedia.org/wiki/Biological_functions_of_nitric_oxide

[149] Victor W.T. Liu, Paul L. Huang (2007). Cardiovascular roles of nitric oxide: A review of insights from nitric oxide synthase gene disrupted mice. *European Society of Cardiology, Cardiovascular Research, 3 January 2008*. doi: http://dx.doi.org/10.1016/j.cardiores.2007.06.024 19-29

[150] Luciano Bernardi, Peter Sleight, Gabriele Bandinelli, Simone Cencetti, Lamberto Fattorini Johanna Wdowczyc-Szulc Alfonso Lagi (2014). *BMJ. 2001 Dec 22; 323(7327): 1446–1449*. Effect of rosary prayer and yoga mantras on autonomic cardiovascular rhythms: comparative study. PMCID: PMC61046 http://www.ncbi.nlm.nih.gov/pmc/articles/PMC61046/

[151] Hummer RA, Rogers RG, Nam CB, Ellison CG.(1999). Religious involvement and U.S. adult mortality. *Demography. 1999 May;36(2):273-85*. PMID: 10332617 http://www.ncbi.nlm.nih.gov/pubmed/10332617

[152] Lin IM, Tai LY, Fan SY (2014). Breathing at a rate of 5.5 breaths per minute with equal inhalation-to-exhalation ratio increases heart rate variability. [Abstract]. *Int J Psychophysiol. 2014 Mar;91(3):206-11*. doi: 10.1016/j.ijpsycho.2013.12.006. PMID: 24380741 http://www.ncbi.nlm.nih.gov/pubmed/24380741

[153] Heart Rate Variability. Wikipedia. Retrieved August 14, 2015 from https://en.wikipedia.org/wiki/Heart_rate_variability

[154] Sztajzel J (2004). Heart rate variability: a noninvasive electrocardiographic method to measure the autonomic nervous system. *Swiss Med Wkly. 2004 Sep 4;134(35-36):514-22*. PMID: 15517504 http://www.ncbi.nlm.nih.gov/pubmed/15517504

[155] Postural orthostatic tachycardia syndrome, Wikipedia. Retreived June 28, 2015 from https://en.wikipedia.org/wiki/Postural_orthostatic_tachycardia_syndrome

[156] Ibid https://en.wikipedia.org/wiki/Postural_orthostatic_tachycardia_syndrome

[157] Postural Tachycardia Syndrome (POTS). Retrieved June 28, 2015 from Physiopedia http://www.physio-pedia.com/Postural_Tachycardia_Syndrome_(POTS)

[158] Underlying Causes of Dysautonomia. Retrieved June 28, 2015 from Dysautonomia International http://www.dysautonomiainternational.org/page.php?ID=150

[159] Benjamin D. Levine, Julie H. Zuckerman, James A. Pawelczyk (1997). Cardiac Atrophy After Bed-Rest Deconditioning, A Nonneural Mechanism for Orthostatic Intolerance. *Circulation, Articles 1997, February 11*. Retrieved June 28, 2015 from http://circ.ahajournals.org/content/96/2/517.long

[160] Underlying Causes of Dysautonomia. Retrieved June 28, 2015 from Dysautonomia International http://www.dysautonomiainternational.org/page.php?ID=150

[161] Sheldon G. Sheps, M.D., High Blood Pressure (hypertension). Mayo Clinic, expert answers. Retrieved June 28, 2015 from http://www.mayoclinic.org/diseases-conditions/high-blood-pressure/expert-answers/pulse-pressure/faq-20058189

[162] Pulse Pressure. Wikipedia. Retrieved June 28, 2015 from https://en.wikipedia.org/wiki/Pulse_pressure

[163] Carolyn Williams, Bronwyn A Kingwell, Kevin Burke, Jane McPherson, and Anthony M Dart (2005). Folic acid supplementation for 3 wk reduces pulse pressure and large artery stiffness independent of MTHFR genotype. *Am J Clin Nutr 2005, February 22*. http://ajcn.nutrition.org/content/82/1/26.full

[164] Peter A. van Zwieten (2001). Drug treatment of isolated systolic hypertension. *Nephrol.Dial.Transplant.(2001) 16 (6): 1095-1097*. doi: 10.1093/ndt/16.6.1095 http://ndt.oxfordjournals.org/content/16/6/1095.full

[165] Peters R, Beckett N, Fagard R, Thijs L, Wang JG, Forette F, Pereira L, Fletcher A, Bulpitt C (2013). Increased pulse pressure linked to dementia: further results from the Hypertension in the Very Elderly Trial – HYVET..*J Hypertens. 2013 Sep;31(9):1868-75*. doi: 10.1097/HJH.0b013e3283622cc6. PMID: 23743809 http://www.ncbi.nlm.nih.gov/pubmed/23743809

[166] Pulse Pressure, Wikipedia. Retrieved June 28, 2015 from https://en.wikipedia.org/wiki/Pulse_pressure

[167] Heavy Periods (menorrhagia). Retrieved June 28, 2015 from NHS Choices http://www.nhs.uk/conditions/Periods-heavy/Pages/Introduction.aspx

[168] Prevalence and Incidence of Anemia. Right Diagnosis, Retrieved June 28, 2015 from http://www.rightdiagnosis.com/a/anemia/prevalence.htm

[169] S. Killip, J. Bennett, M.D. Chambers (2007). Iron Deficiency Anemia, *Am Fam Physician. 2007 Mar 1;75(5):671-678*; http://www.aafp.org/afp/2007/0301/p671.html

[170] M. Wessling-Resnick Annu (2010).Iron Homeostasis and the Inflammatory Response. *Annu Rev Nutr. 2010 Aug 21; 30: 105–122*. doi: 10.1146/annurev.nutr.012809.104804 PMC3108097 http://www.ncbi.nlm.nih.gov/pmc/articles/PMC3108097/

[171] The American Association of Immunologists. Arthur Fernandez Coca, M.D. (1875–1959) Brief Bio. Retrieved August 17, 2015 from https://www.aai.org/About/History/Notable_Members/The_JI/Coca_Arthur.html

[172] A. F. Coca (1956). The Pulse Test. Retrieved June 30, 2015 from http://www.soilandhealth.org/02/0201hyglibcat/020108.coca.pdf

[173] A. F. Coca (1956). The Pulse Test. Retrieved June 30, 2015 from http://www.soilandhealth.org/02/0201hyglibcat/020108.coca.pdf

[174] K. Alagiakrishnan (2007). Postural and Postprandial Hypotension: Approach to Management. *Geriatrics and Aging. 2007;10(5):298-304*. http://www.medscape.com/viewarticle/559578_5

Made in the USA
Middletown, DE
10 August 2017